Pain, Anxiety, and Grief

PAIN, ANXIETY, AND GRIEF

PHARMACOTHERAPEUTIC CARE OF THE DYING PATIENT AND THE BEREAVED

**Ivan K. Goldberg,
Austin H. Kutscher,
and Sidney Malitz,**
editors

with the assistance of
Lillian G. Kutscher

Columbia University Press
New York
1986

Library of Congress Cataloging in Publication Data
Main entry under title:

Pain, anxiety, and grief.

(Columbia University Press/Foundation of Thanatology series)
Includes bibliographies and index.
1. Terminal care. 2. Bereavement. 3. Pain—Chemotherapy. 4. Anxiety—Chemotherapy. 5. Grief. 6. Neuropsychopharmacology. I. Goldberg, Ivan K., 1934– . II. Kutscher, Austin H. III. Malitz, Sidney, 1923– . IV. Series. [DNLM: 1. Anxiety—drug therapy. 2. Pain—drug therapy. 3. Palliative Treatment. 4. Terminal Care. WB 310 P144]
R726.8.P34   1985   616'.029   85-9685
Library of Congress Cataloging in Publication Data
ISBN 0-231-04742-8 (alk. paper)

Columbia University Press
New York   Guildford, Surrey
Copyright © 1986 Columbia University Press
All rights reserved

Printed in the United States of America

This book is Smyth-sewn and printed on permanent and durable acid-free paper

Contents

Preface vii

Acknowledgment ix

I. Practical, Ethical, and Moral Issues Relating to Pharmacotherapy

1. General Systems Approach to the Psychopharmacologic Treatment of the Dying Patient
   IRWIN M. GREENBERG   3
2. The Needs of Dying Patients STEWART G. WOLF   15
3. Practical and Philosophical Concepts of Pain Control
   WILLIAM REGELSON   19
4. Some Limits of Psychotropic Drugs in Supportive Treatment of Oncology Patients
   PATRICIA MURRAY   28
5. Psychological Hazards of Drug Therapy
   RICHARD S. BLACHER   34
6. Drugs, Physicians, and Patients IRVING S. WRIGHT   38
7. Problems of Polypharmacy DAVID M. BENJAMIN   41
8. Suicide by Drug Overdose BRUCE L. DANTO   53

II. Controlling the Dying Patient's Pain

9. Pain Control in the Treatment of Cancer
   IVAN K. GOLDBERG   65
10. The Use of Diamorphine in the Management of Terminal Cancer (*Historical amd Chronological Evolution, 1971*) ROBERT G. TWYCROSS   70
11. The Use and Abuse of Narcotic Analgesics in Terminal Cancer (*Historical and Chronological Evolution, 1974*) ROBERT G. TWYCROSS   79
12. Continuing and Terminal Care—Overview of Analgesia (*Historical and Chronological Evolution, 1978*) ROBERT G. TWYCROSS   105

13. Cancer Pain: A Comparison of Methadone,
Methadone-Cocaine, and Methadone-Amphetamine
MICHAEL WEINTRAUB, AMY VALENTINE AND
STEPHEN STECKEL   128

14. Utility of a Combination of Stimulant Drugs
with Opiates in the Production of Analgesia
WAYNE O. EVANS   142

15. Pharmacokinetic Aspects of Analgesia During
Palliative Care M. KEERI-SZANTO   148

16. Relief for the Dying and the Bereaved: The Role
of Psychopharmacologic Agents and Analgesics
CHING-PIAU CHIEN, BALU KALAYAM, AND
REUBEN J. SILVER   151

17. The Cancer Ward IRENE B. SEELAND   159

18. Pharmacologic Agents—Barriers or Tools?
SAMUEL C. KLAGSBRUN   164

19. Psychological Responses in the Dying Patient:
A Role for Behaviorally Active Peptide Hormones?
DANIEL CARR   169

III. Relieving the Grief and Anxiety of Bereavement

20. Acute Grief: A Physician's Viewpoint
ROBERT G. TWYCROSS   177

21. Psychopharmacologic Treatment of Bereavement
ROBERT KELLNER, RICHARD T. RADA, AND
WALTER W. WINSLOW   185

22. Tricyclic Antidepressants in the Treatment
of Depression in Conjugal Bereavement: A Controlled
Study PHILIP R. MUSKIN AND ARTHUR RIFKIN   200

23. The Relevance of Psychopharmacologic Agents
for the Bereaved in a Community Mental Health
Center (CMHC) ARLEEN I. SKVERSKY, RICHARD F.
TISLOW, AND ANTHONY F. SANTORE   210

Index   215

Preface

The advances in medical technology that have transformed life-threatening diseases into long-term, chronic illnesses have yet to deal definitively with the pain and anxiety of the dying patient and the grief of the bereaved. Although the costs of protracted illness are now measured in terms of dollars and cents, allocation of resources, and decreases in the social productivity of individuals, they have a different significance when extension of life means extension of suffering. In most life-threatening illness, pain and discomfort eventually impose a toll that affects the quality of life of those, including both patients and their family members, who have benefited—until the quest for cure has become unrealistic.

Few would deny that, within the modalities offered the critically ill to ease suffering, there is a broad range of pharmacotherapeutic agents. But many would question how and when these drugs are currently prescribed and administered. The British have introduced us to the hospice philosophy of total care for the terminally ill patient—total care embracing the physical, psychosocial, psychological, and spiritual nurturing of an individual until the very end of life. If we have been impressed enough to attempt to transplant the hospice system from the Old World to our shores, many are still reluctant to make the fullest necesssary use of the psychopharmacologic armamentarium as "fail safe" final measures to ease the passage of the dying.

In this book, the pioneer work of Dr. Robert G. Twycross at St. Christopher's Hospice in London has been chronicled in several chapters of historical import. Regrettably, for all the good intentions and high standards of our pain control experts, the taboos against appropriate usage of narcotics and other agents even for the care of the terminal patient have not been eradicated and we have yet to eliminate our fears of these as uncontrollable social hazards and substances of the highest abuse potential. Although testimony is presented in this text on behalf of the effectiveness of those drugs that are already accepted in our pharmacopoeias, many question whether these drugs are used properly, in sufficient quantity, and at appropriate time intervals.

As those who have shared in this effort acknowledge, pain is more than a physical phenomenon: it is a complex of physical, psychosocial, psychological, and spiritual disorders. Nor is there any panacea capable of obliterating all of the suffering it causes, although much relief has been achieved when caregivers have cared enough. The thrust of pain emerges from different sources and in different degrees as it confronts the dying and the bereaved. That thoughtful, caring scientists are still not completely satisfied with what they can offer patients, that they are constantly seeking new ways to understand the phenomena of pain, that they continue to search for new concepts of pain dynamics and management as well as new agents to accomplish the tasks—these are the messages conveyed in this book.

Experience demonstrates that controlling the pain of the dying and easing the grief and anxiety of the bereaved are issues of practical, ethical, and moral significance. Experience also assures us that what has been accomplished by our most diligent researchers, academicians, and clinicians serves as a base for future discoveries. What science gains, it rarely loses. So, as it has come to pass that advances have been made in medical technology and disease control, it should some day come to pass that death can be confronted with dignity and bereavement borne with hopefulness.

The Editors

Acknowledgment

The editors wish to acknowledge the support and encouragement of the Foundation of Thanatology in the preparation of this volume. All royalties from the sale of this book are assigned to the Foundation of Thanatology, a tax exempt, not for profit, public, scientific and educational foundation.

Thanatology, a new subspecialty of medicine, is involved in scientific and humanistic inquiries and the application of the knowledge derived therefrom to the subjects of the psychological aspects of dying; reactions to loss, death, and grief; and recovery from bereavement.

The Foundation of Thanatology is dedicated to promoting enlightened health care for life-threatened or terminally ill patients and their families. The Foundation's orientation is a positive one based on the philosophy of fostering a more mature understanding of life-threatening illness, the problems of grief, and the more effective and humane management and treatment of patients and family members in times of crisis.

Pain, Anxiety, and Grief

I.
PRACTICAL, ETHICAL, AND MORAL ISSUES RELATING TO PHARMACOTHERAPY

1.
GENERAL SYSTEMS APPROACH TO THE PSYCHOPHARMACOLOGIC TREATMENT OF THE DYING PATIENT

Irwin M. Greenberg

During the past two decades, there has been a noticeable shift in the effort made by psychiatry, medicine, and allied fields to deal with the intrapsychic and interpersonal aspects of the phenomenon of death. Much of the effort has gone into psychotherapeutic intervention with the dying patients and their families, principally with people who had not had previous psychiatric illness. Although relatively little was done systematically with respect to use of psychopharmacologic agents in treatment of the elements of the social system comprising the dying patient's family, the groundwork for such investigation was laid by overt expressions of alterations in value system. Stated otherwise, an axiom of principle appears to have been stated by those dealing with the psychosocial problems of the dying person—that there indeed existed a valid field of study in the psychological treatment of the dying patient. In retrospect, this was a radical departure from the classical concerns of both the psychodynamic and biological schools of thought. The former, influenced strongly by Freud's emphasis, assiduously avoided the problem of death as a thing in itself. The latter was much more concerned with the metabolic, electrophysiological, and genetic processes underlying defined psychiatric disease.

It is not appropriate to mention here, more than in passing, a few of the many possible reasons for this shift in the spirit of the times with respect to the treatment of dying people. The unusual widespread violence throughout all of the world since the beginning of this century has been an unavoidable fact to be faced by all. Those who would choose not to think of death if they could were literally coerced to do so. As the world changed politically after 1950, the human needs of many people who had hitherto been ignored or considered exploitable began changing rapidly. The death or misery of those distant from us in space or background became less deniable. With these two phenomena of widespread violence and the new egalitarianism there arose a new attitude toward religion and death in many diversified ethnic and socioeconomic groups. Salvation, whether by grace or works, appeared less possible and existentialism increased in popularity, even to those who had never heard of it.

As a consequence of these three interrelated changes—one of action, one of thought, and one of feeling—there arose a change of attitude among a few workers in the biomedical and social science professions. This attitudinal change allowed these few to seek the capability to treat death as an aspect of life. There followed the discovery of new, or the rediscovery of old, methods of treating dying patients and their families.

As the capability to treat such people appeared, some work was described by Eissler (1955), Shneidman and Farberow (1957), Feifel (1959), Greenberg (1964), and Greenberg and Alexander (1962). Eissler was one of the first psychiatrists to describe treatment of the dying patient. Shneidman and Farberow were interested principally in suicide. Feifel worked with a multidisciplinary approach, and Greenberg investigated reunion fantasies. Some of the helpful earlier concepts of Grotjahn (1960) and Zilboorg (1943) were rediscovered in terms of the recognition of mortality as an important intrapsychic matter. The questioning of older attitudes toward the dying person grew, and Kübler-Ross's (1969, 1975) ideas were very well disseminated. Death, which was becoming more depersonalized with advances in technology, was repersonalized through efforts such as hers. So widespread has the awareness of the need to treat the dying person become (Becker 1973; GAP 1975) that even courses for preparation of Psychiatric Board Examinations provide equal time for this subject.

A Theoretical Approach

With increasing awareness of the need for psychological treatment of the dying patient and the family, interest in psychopharmacologic agents for these people also grew, but with systematization.

Death clearly presents many physiological, as well as psychological and familial, problems. The treatment of all in a systematic manner, lending appropriate emphasis to one aspect or another of intervention, required a more general theory than those used by workers in the field. Von Bertalanffy's General Systems Theory (1975) would appear to be a suitable framework for developing such a theory, and it is this point that the remainder of this presentation develops. The development includes a description of a form of General Systems Theory, with emphasis on the recognition of primary and secondary subsystem dysfunction as differentiated from *critical* subsystem dysfunction. The concept is demonstrated to imply that treatment may at times be directed to factors other than those of primary etiology (Greenberg 1978). Clinical examples of such a formulation are described for patients who are *not* dying, as well as for the dying patient, particularly with reference to use of psychotropic medication.

The role of the influence of social ideology is also reviewed, for it appears to enter into treatment decisions wittingly or otherwise. The necessity for clinicians to deal with their own ideology and with those of others is demonstrated to be of paramount importance and indeed to constitute one of the most critical parts of the treatment process.

General Systems Theory

A brief description of von Bertalanffy's theory begins with the a priori assumption that any given organization of a living organism or set of organisms may be taken as an index system. For conventional purposes, the individual human being may be taken as the index system in this discussion. The classical anatomic and physiological approaches then have the organism's subsystems defined by their functions—for example, musculoskeletal, cardiovascular, hematopoietic, central nervous systems. The classical approach then defines subsystems by organ, tissue, cell, organelles, enzyme systems, and molecular species. In neuropsychiatry, a subdivision of the central nervous system is often used, as is done later in this discussion.

In classical psychological and sociological theories, the human organism is usually considered as an element of the nuclear family system and extended family system, as well as of a more extensive interpersonal field system and of the society-at-large. The last usually includes the other systems as subsystems but may represent an anomie-generating structure for certain reference—that is, sociocultural groups or social classes. In some societies, there is a well-defined relationship between the reference group and society-at-large systems on the one hand and caste structure and function on the other.

In using a General Systems approach, it is best to consider first the anatomic or structural intactness of each subsystem or supersystem, be it a biological or social entity. For example, is there a broken home or disrupted nuclear family, or is there myocardial damage in the cardiovascular system? Secondly, function should be considered. Is the structurally intact nuclear family functioning as a family, or is it one in which communication and affective interchange are at a minimum? Similarly, is an anatomically intact organ actually functioning, or is there a loss of function? Thirdly, the quality of function should be investigated. Does a nuclear family provide optimal care and support to its members or does it only carry out motions? Does the cardiac output meet the requirements of the organism? Does the social support system really provide adequate insurance? Many other examples can be constructed at any level of system organization.

Fourthly, the time relationships of each system must be considered. Such considerations range, for example, from peristaltic activity or respiratory rate under different conditions to the long-term evolution of a nuclear family or social group.

In addition to the considerations of structure, function, quality, and time in each subsystem, there is the additional dimension of the *interactions between* systems. These interactional processes are of as great a significance as the systems themselves. The interactional processes also require examination of structure, function, quality, and time relations. Subsystems within the same system may interact, as in peristaltic activity following a meal. Moreover, subsystems may interact across systems, as in the respiratory compensation for metabolic acidosis or alkalosis. In family function, one member may become the active one to support the illness of another. Social systems—for example, day-care centers for children—may develop to replace dysfunctional or structurally absent extended families.

In dealing with the use of psychotropic medication, it is necessary to inquire into the subsystems of the central nervous system and their interactions. Many, but not all, of these structures of the central nervous system were defined a century ago. Some were functionally defined only recently. The interaction between subsystems as implemented by neurotransmitters is currently undergoing extensive investigation.

For the purposes of the neuropsychiatrist, the great classical cerebellar and rolandic sensory-motor subsystems hold the least interest; they are the purview of the neurologist. Of much greater interest are (1) the great subcortical structures; (2) the temporal-parietal sensory, cognitive, and integrative structures; and (3) the great frontal-prefrontal organized motor conceptual structures. Many of the functions of these great cortical neuropsychological subsystems have been described by Luria (1973). However, the subcortical structures are very frequently those that the clinical psychiatrist must also understand. Essentially, aside from the extrapyramidal motoric system, these reduce to the reticular and limbic systems. The former exerts its influence by activation, inhibition, and integration. The latter deals with emotion, olfaction, recent memory, and hormone metabolism and, by means of the hypothalamus, acts as the upper motor neuron center for autonomic functions.

Clinical neuropsychiatrists, then, deal with reticular, limbic, intrapsychic, familial, and interpersonal interaction systems. It is always necessary for them to discover which is of primary etiological importance and which is of critical importance for intervention. It is also necessary to ensure the significance of the presence or absence of other system dysfunction.

Primary system dysfunction refers to basic etiology. For example, myocardial infarction is often secondary to arteriosclerotic coronary artery disease. The ensuing heart failure is, in turn, secondary to myocardial insufficiency. Treatment, however, is aimed at relief of pain and reduction of the heart's workload by reducing fluid volume. The latter constitutes *critical* system intervention. Similarly, partial complex seizures of temporal lobe epilepsy may result from repeated febrile cerebral insult. The primary system dysfunction lies within the irritable electrical focus and is treatable with anticonvulsant medication. The *critical* system dysfunction may lie in the family system and in obtaining agreement from the family that the patient indeed has the disease we think is present. Thus, the practice of clinical psychopharmacology is often aimed not only at the primary or etiological system dysfunction; it is often directed, in addition, to the familial or intrapsychic systems, which often reflect attitudes toward illness.

Of frequent importance is the matter of side effects, which may be consciously more distressing to the patient than the original illness. It would be difficult to obtain therapeutic compliance for chlorpromazine from a sign painter exposed to the sun. It would be equally difficult to obtain cooperation from a watch repairman who developed tremors with fluphenazine. There are, of course, highly idiosyncratic familial responses to side effects, such as parental objection to nasal congestion in an aggressive child treated with thioridazine.

What may be of greater importance in all these cases is the internalized value system, which is here considered to correspond internally to what Erikson has called ego-identity (1950). The propensity to deny the need for medication is extremely common among people who have learned that doing things for oneself is one of the greatest of good things. The belief in freedom of the will is, at times, so great that patients with frank seizure disorder or metabolic illness such as diabetes find it extremely difficult to face imperfections in their organisms and believe in their ability to do everything themselves. There is the additional negative value attached to the need for dependency, even when realistic, in these people.

The *critical* system dysfunction, then, becomes one of attitudes and belief, both in the patient and in the nuclear family in many instances. Such beliefs are widespread and culturally reinforced in the Western world.

Application of the Theory in Treatment of Dying Patients and Their Families

The assessment of critical system dysfunction in the case of a dying patient often extends beyond evaluation of the patient and the bereaved to the treatment team. As an example, a case is cited:

> The patient was an upper-middle-class housewife of Mediterranean ancestry with advanced pulmonary carcinoma for whom psychiatric evaluation was requested to ascertain whether a spinothalamic tractotomy for pain relief was psychiatrically reasonable. In the referral request, the question was raised concerning the possibility of "trouble at home" precipitating an episode of excessive reaction to pain. There was no evidence of cerebral metastasis. On interview, the patient appeared to be a remarkably intact woman who understood the nature of her disease and who appeared to be using every resource to remain alive. There was no evidence of hysteria or other functional disorder, nor was there evidence of cerebral dysfunction. There was no indication of "trouble at home" or of *la belle indifference*. Interview with visitors corroborated the impression given by examination of the patient. The consultant's opinion was that the patient was functioning well intrapsychically and interpersonally and that there was no psychiatric contraindication to the operation. However, the patient died three days later.

It was evident, on system analysis, that the primary system dysfunction was directly related to the anatomic and systemic effects of a spreading carcinoma, which, in turn, was causing pain, and because of which the patient died. The critical system dysfunction was, however, to be found in an important element of the social system—namely, in the treatment team. It is excellent practice for a neurosurgeon not to operate if there is a possibility of equally effective nonsurgical—that is, medical or psychiatric—treatment. Thus the *value system* of the neurosurgeon who requested the consultation came to the forefront. Moreover, the discrepancy between the surgeon's view of appropriate reaction to pain and the actual reaction of the patient was evident; this discrepancy might best be described as arising from cultural differences. Lastly, the neurosurgical service in question was a research service dealing principally with temporal lobe disorders and one that was not accustomed to dealing with dying patients. As a consequence, the advanced stage of the patient's illness was not easily recognized. The interaction of all three factors led to the request for psychiatric consultation.

Further system analysis of this case would reveal that not only was there a cultural difference between the patient and the surgeon but also there was an even more significant reference group difference between the patient and the usual patient population with which the surgeon dealt. He was simply not used to dealing with dying patients in pain, nor was the rest of the staff. It is not surprising that the ordinary method of denial of death came into play here.

Thus, the essential point illustrated by the case is the need to explore the acceptance of the patient's death by treating staff. It is very difficult for physicians, nurses, and others to accept the pain, malaise, fear, anxiety, and depression of the dying patient when there is not yet recognition that the patient is indeed dying. Once there is the recognition, on the part of the social system—that is, the treatment staff—that the patient is dying, there should be such recognition on the part of the family. A form of psychotherapeutic intervention should occur in the staff's interactions with the patient's family to enable family members and other bereaved people to handle their own, as well as the patient's feelings. If indicated, psychotropic medication may be prescribed for the bereaved.

If there is indeed recognition of impending death by both staff and family, several new issues must be addressed, the first of which is to ascertain the meaning of death to the patient and to essential staff and family members involved. In many instances, a family physician, clergyman, or close friend can be very helpful in answering the questions for the patient and for some family member. In other instances the clinician will have to find out *de novo*.

Among some important attitudes toward death are those dealing with punishment for sin and with belief in salvation, predestination, and reunion in the hereafter. Although it is evident that the patient's beliefs are of paramount importance, it is also important to deal with family and staff beliefs. These beliefs strongly influence the choice of medication, psychotropic and otherwise, to be administered to the patient.

As stated previously, the principal symptoms, other than those of delirium or of chronic brain syndrome, in the psychiatrically intact dying patient are pain, malaise, anxiety, and depression. These symptoms are usually treatable to some degree *if they are recognized* as *treatable* symptoms. Probably pain is the most distressing of all symptoms to a dying person. Frequently both anxiety and depression are relieved when pain is relieved. The use of analgesics, narcotics, and tricyclic antidepressant agents is often indicated for pain. The questions of amount and frequency of dosage are sometimes of greater importance than the actual choice of medication. It is here that the value system of staff influences the treatment regimen.

1. If there is denial of the patient's nearness to death, there is also the great possibility of denial of pain.
2. If there is acknowledgment of the patient's nearness to death, the unconscious values of belief in punishment for sin and the moral value of suffering may influence staff members to avoid using appropriate medication.
3. If there is neither denial nor *conscious* belief in puritanical morality, there may be an unrealistic expectation on the part of staff, and possibly of family, for independence on the part of the patient. This may appear clinically as concern not to allow the patient to become "dependent" on medication and is often as not rooted in cognitive confusion. Such confusion equates a dying, often elderly, person with a younger drug-dependent person with entirely different problems.

Here the Western ethic of independence at any cost interferes with appropriate treatment.

4. If there *is* recognition of the need for medication, there may be insufficient dosage or frequency because of lack of awareness of the time effectiveness of dosage. For example, the maximum effective time for some analgesic or narcotic agents may wear off within *three*, and not four hours, so that it might be much wiser to administer the medication every three hours.

To recapitulate, medication administration may not be optimal, because of (1) intrapsychic reasons (for example, denial); (2) value system reason (for example, belief in punitive morality); (3) cognitive confusion (for example, lack of recognition of the difference between drug dependency in the dying patient and in the younger, physically healthy patient); (4) incomplete knowledge (as in the failure to recognize optimal activity levels of analgesic drugs).

There are, indeed, some patients who might prefer to experience pain if the treatment of such pain reduces their cognitive and relational capacities. Even in these cases, when the clinician has ascertained that the patient is not complying with conscious or unconscious staff or family demands, both pharmacologic and psychological interventions are possible. For example, diphenylhydantoin may alter peripheral nerve conduction, as well as alter thalamic conduction, and thus relieve pain sensation without inducing loss of awareness. It may be particularly useful in conjunction with tricyclic antidepresent medication. Hypnosis may often be of benefit to reduce pain in suitable patients, so that no medication may be appropriate at times.

To return to the pharmacologic treatment of family and other bereaved people, it is very important to bear in mind that such people are not always psychiatrically intact but may suffer from any psychiatric disorder simply by chance. Simple reassurance, supportive psychotherapy, and the use of anxiolytic agents (GAP 1975) will not always be helpful. It is necessary to assess the psychiatric status of any important family member and treat accordingly. Such prompt intervention may abort severe neurotic depression or even prevent psychotic episodes. Again it is necessary to recognize that death is imminent to a loved one and that such a loss may often act as a precipitant to psychiatric decompensation.

Free Will and Calvinism

In an effort to help the clinician deal with the effect of family and staff value systems on the pharmacologic treatment of the dying patient, a few words should be said about dominant Western tradition in the matter.

In dealing with the issue of death as punishment for sin, it is essential to recall that this was a pervasive theme of the Middle Ages, is found mentioned in Hamlet, when the ghost tells the prince to leave his mother to Heaven; and is not uncommonly found in the religious backgrounds of people in our own day. An awareness of this belief, especially in terms of sin's being a product of free will, may be very helpful clinically in dealing with seemingly punitive staff and family. Similarly, classical Calvinism holds that we all must carry out God's will and that suffering has been preordained, especially for those who are not members of the Elect. In such cases, staff or family will appear resistant to the use of medication for relief of suffering, fearing a violation of what has been preordained. Again, awareness of the possibility of this belief may make it a good deal easier to discuss the matter and have the patient treated appropriately. These beliefs are often unconscious and may be as deeply rooted as any infantile conflictual material. A nonjudgmental question concerning them may often allow treatment to progress.

Summary and Conclusion

This discussion has presented a General Systems Theory approach to the pharmacologic treatment of the dying patient, the family, and other bereaved people. It has assumed that such pharmacologic treatment, especially for pain, is often appropriate and necessary. It has further examined the nature of belief systems of family and staff, within a systems framework, emphasizing the effect that value systems and other intrapsychic and social beliefs have on the patient's treatment. It is suggested that discussion of such beliefs with staff and family may allow the clinician more freedom in treating the patient pharmacologically and may ensure greater cooperation from those concerned.

References

Becker, E. 1973, *The Denial of Death*. New York: The Free Press.
Eissler, K. R. 1955. *The Psychiatrist and the Dying Patient*. New York: International Universities Press.
Erikson, E. H. 1950. *Childhood and Society*. New York: Norton.
Feifel, H., ed. 1959. *The Meaning of Death*. New York: McGraw-Hill.
Greenberg, I. M., n.d. In John A. Talbot, ed. *Social Calvinism, Free Will, Ideology and Treatment in State Hospitals: Problems and Potentials*. New York: Human Sciences Press.
―――― 1978. "General Systems Theory: Social and Biological Interactions." *Psychiatry*.
Greenberg, I. M. and I. E. Alexander. 1962. "Some Correlates of Thoughts and Feelings Concerning Death." *Hillside Hospital Journal* 2:120–26.
Grotjahn, M. 1960. "Ego Identity and the Fear of Death and Dying." *Hillside Hospital Journal* 9:147–55.
Group for the Advancement of Psychiatry (GAP) Committee on Research. 1975. *Pharmacotherapy and Psychotherapy: Paradoxes, Problems and Progress*. New York: Group for the Advancement of Psychiatry 9, Report 93 (March).
Hinton J. 1967. *Dying*. Harmondsworth, Middlesex: Penguin Books.
Kübler-Ross, E. 1969. *On Death and Dying*. New York: Macmillan.
Kübler-Ross, E., ed. 1975. *Death, the Final Stage of Growth*. Englewood Cliffs, N.J.: Prentice-Hall.
Luria, A. R. 1973. *The Working Brain*. New York: Basic Books.
Shneidman, E. S. and N. L. Farberow. 1957. *Clues to Suicide*. New York: McGraw-Hill.
Von Bertalanffy, L. 1975. *Perspectives on General System Theory*. New York: Brazilier.
Zilboorg, G. 1943. "Fear of Death." *Psychoanalytic Quarterly* 12:465–75.

2.
THE NEEDS OF DYING PATIENTS

Stewart G. Wolf

Dealing with dying patients involves more than relieving their pain; comfort and serenity, in a dying patient experiencing pain, depend on more than blunting the pain. So, while management of pain is very important, there are other objectives. These fall into several categories: the need to blunt depression and obsessive ruminative thinking; the need to reduce tension; the need to weaken barriers—between patient and doctor, and patient and family—the need for interhuman communications, especially when the precious time for this communication is running out; the need to induce serenity and detachment. No drug substitutes for the warm, understanding support of the physician, and time has a physiological component and is not simply a way of repressing feelings.

The power of the relationship between patient and physician can be illustrated when measurable aspects of the body physiology are modified. In this instance, I have selected nausea because it is easier to document than pain. In nausea, we have an associated physiologic change that can be measured by a relaxation of the stomach (so that it hangs loosely like a bag) and by an increase of the contractual state of the duodenum, which makes a reverse gradient and pushes whatever is in the small intestine back toward the stomach. In an experimental setup for one patient, a three-lumen tube was put down the patient's throat. Gastric contractions were recorded. At first, not much was happening in the stomach, and there were duodenal contractions measurable through the second lumen. The third lumen was open so that whatever we wanted could be introduced into the stomach or gastric juice withdrawn from it. The tip of the tube was in the first portion of the duodenum. Then, nausea was induced by a commonly reliable mechanism—running warm water into one ear and cold water into another. The nausea was associated with a sensation of whatever motor activity was going on in the stomach, a decrease in the tone of the stomach as it hung loose; in the duodenum it was associated with an increase in the contractual state and a regurgitation of an inserted balloon that carried the tube back toward the stomach. No matter how nausea is induced, this is the physiological effect.

With a particular subject, after the lumen tube was in place, we undertook a discussion about pregnancy. Actually, this woman was not pregnant, but we simply discussed the possibility. In association with this, her gastric activity ceased, her duodenum activity increased, and the tube was regurgitated back toward the stomach. This is a clear illustration of what can happen in a relationship with respect to measurable physiologic change.

We became very interested in studying the nausea and vomiting of pregnancy. The gastric motor activity in an individual who was subject to the nausea and vomiting of pregnancy but who did not happen to be nauseated at the time was recorded.

Gastric contractions were taking place. When we introduced a 10-cc solution of syrup of ipecac through the open lumen, gastric activity ceased within five minutes and the individual said that she was nauseated. After a time the effects of the ipecac wore off, the stomach was contracting again, and the nausea was gone.

This patient was asked to return to the laboratory on a day when she was nauseous. We could perceive no vigorous motor activity in the stomach at all. At this point, I told the patient that we had just received a shipment of a new medicine that eliminated nausea. I injected the same 10-cc of ipecac down the open lumen of her tube. Instead of becoming more nauseous, the woman reported that her nausea had gone, and we recorded a return of gastric contractions.

This particular experiment illustrates a number of things, among them the enormous power of the doctor-patient situation and the fact that this power exceeds that of ordinarily powerful pharmacodynamic agents. In a parallel experiment with patients who were experiencing pain of several weeks' duration following abdominal surgery, we introduced a "new medicine," "a special shipment from Germany," which was "far more powerful as a pain killer than morphine but did not have any toxicity, did not cause constipation, did not have any of the side effects produced by morphine." The bottles were carefully marked and the nurses were cautioned about not getting them mixed up. For those individuals who were given the usual postoperative medication—15 mm of morphine, q4h prn—we substituted this "special medicine." These individuals were able to call for injections whenever they wanted. The result, perhaps, could have been anticipated. The special medicine was just saline solution, and the patients who received it did much better and had less pain than those patients who were receiving morphine. When we talked with them and revealed what had been done, the general reply was that the thing that had helped most was to be able to ring the buzzer and get the medicine right away. The frustrating thing was to be in pain, call the nurse, and have the nurse say, "I'm sorry, but you have another hour and fifteen minutes to wait before another shot is due."

New developments in pain research offer the possibility of important drug and nondrug solutions for dealing with patients in pain. The issue is not just one of interfering with incoming pain "traffic" but also of recruiting a central nervous system mechanism that actually modulates, damps, and restricts that incoming pain traffic. Indirect evidence on the existence of such a system goes back quite a long time, but only in the past eight to ten years has the evidence evolved to the point that we are quite sure it is there. We know something about how it works, especially about the lower levels of the nervous system; we still have a great deal to learn about the higher levels.

For a long time there was a dispute about whether pain was carried in its own system of neurons or whether any neuron can carry pain. As so often occurs in medical controversy, everyone was right. There are some effluent neurons capable of carrying various kinds of sensations from the periphery, presumably because of different kinds of coating, but there are also central nervous system neurons in the dorsal horn that are specialists and carry only pain.

However, in addition to knowledge about the physiology of pain, we must recognize the importance of social management of the patient in pain. The effect of the social setting has been demonstrated in experiments with alcohol. Laboratory workers given enormous amounts of alcohol in the laboratory really could not get very drunk. The social circumstances probably were not conducive to that. Even more important, no matter what was mixed together and consumed, we could not produce hangovers. So social circumstances are useful in the management of the patient. There is no cookbook approach, for every patient is an individual.

What is to be done for a patient who has had pain for a long time? There is not anything definitive. It depends on a lot of things that have to do with the patient's identity, goals, vulnerabilities, and so forth. Behavioral modification in groups takes advantage of special peculiarities of people. This approach is not appropriate for some people. They do not like to get into that togetherness, sharing situation. Others, on the other hand, derive enormous support from the sharing experience. It is important not to prescribe something without understanding the patient and the patient's needs.

The physician's job is to relieve and to share the burden. It is not the mission of medicine to defeat death. Similarly, the objective of medicine is not to create a heaven on earth, to keep everybody free of feeling, free of suffering. The Christian and other martyrs have proved that there can be something ennobling about suffering—although we do not recommend emulating this. However, with a sense of worthwhileness and the support—the unique support—that physicians, nurses, and social workers can give, the ability to tolerate a situation, the ability to face a difficult circumstance in life, and the positive aspect of being able to manage oneself in a suffering and uncomfortable position can be an invigorating experience.

3.
PRACTICAL AND PHILOSOPHICAL CONCEPTS OF PAIN CONTROL

William Regelson

There are facts about pain that represent more than its physiology or pathophysiology. In coronary insufficiency, people say that the pain serves as a warning to stop activity, and that makes it good pain. Obviously, pain fulfills a good role from the point of view of mobilization, and it is easy to speak about pain as being beneficial. Yet these are our feelings when *we* do not suffer the pain.

We also have to think about the fact that patients' pain is readily transmitted to the medical staff. In terms of medical management, obviously patients suffering from pain and anxiety in relation to their needs can quickly inflict psychic pain on the people administering to these needs. Then we face an interaction between the medical staff—nurses, doctors, and so forth—and there arises a pattern of interaction between what the patients are asking for or what the patients are signaling with their complaints.

The fact that concerns me most is that for reasons related to our own reactions to the patient, we frequently produce premature death pharmacologically by so heavily sedating patients that they are unable to enjoy or participate in the level of life still remaining. In this regard, we have to be aware of the fact that we are managing two kinds of pain: acute pain—associated with side effects such as changes in pulse, profuse sweating, hypertension and physiological reactions—and chronic pain. In confronting chronic pain in the patient who is chronically ill, we are dealing with what chronic pain does to the personality of the individual, the whole problem of depression, despondency, and despair. If one measures people on psychiatric scales, using the PF 16 or the MMPI or any similar psychometric tests, these individuals are assessed as despondent and depressed. With anyone who is complaining of chronic pain, there is underlying depression and anxiety present constantly. In relieving the anxiety and the depression, of course, physicians play a therapeutic role.

Many physicians become involved in using psychic energizers, with particular emphasis on the tricyclics or the monoamine oxidase inhibitors used to treat the endogenous depressions seen in manic depressives. Some are useful as sedatives for inducing sleep, a use approved by the FDA. However, in dealing with the patient in pain we confront a despondency that is independent of an endogenous depression, that is not a biochemical manic depressive phenomenon but something related to the realistic problem of pain or cancer and related to the quality of life as it reflects feelings of survival: "Am I going to see the next spring? Am I going to survive until next month?" When visitors come, the pattern of interreaction produces a mixed response, and there is real despondency because the person who is dying is giving up something.

This person is not suffering from the depersonalization and psychosis of a true endogenous depression. In my own experience, then, the use of psychic energizers is counterproductive. Although there are cancer patients with preexisting endogenous depressions who can be helped by these agents, applying them without realizing when there is a realistic reason for despondency is using them inappropriately.

Agents we tend to forget about are the amphetamines. Many patients in the terminal phases of life suffer from anorexia, and weight loss is a real problem. We are always trying to encourage appetite, so we forget that amphetamines have analgesic properties that are useful in the relief of pain. They are biphasic in their effects and work on several levels. Although they can enhance sensitivity to pain, after a while a reverse phase occurs and patients have a true analgesic response. Dexedrine, for example, is a psychic energizer that can restore a patient's alertness and interest in what is going on.

The person who gives the medicine is a critical force in a pattern of reinforcement as it relates to the meaning of giving the drug. In other words, a person should never give a drug he does not believe in. For all caregivers there must be a very strong belief system. As a medical oncologist, I never give chemotherapy that I do not believe in. I transmit a belief and I am part of a system. The physicians' white coats or the nurses' uniforms and our belief in the medication that we are giving are absolutely critical. When we give a drug, we are conveying the fact that it is useful. This is very clear and very important, but, unfortunately, because we are living in an age of informed consent, we are forced in effect to defeat our own purpose. We go into the side effects, we go into the negatives, we go into the odds. Now a person like me learns how to play the game according to the law—versus what I consider to be humanistically important and curative for patients. I accentuate the positive in a way that I think is meaningful to the patient in a therapeutic sense. I transmit my belief, and I think this can affect a patient's response because belief is a part of a placebo reaction. The effectiveness of the medicine is increased by doing this.

There are also reinforcing techniques that can be used. For example, when I visit a patient who is suffering from pain despite having received a narcotic shortly before, I often tell the nurse to give the patient an extra dose of narcotic. In this way, I reinforce my role as somebody who can relieve pain and play a dominant role as someone who can help. I use drugs that are pleasant and that reinforce my role as a human being.

Of course, someone might say to me, "What are you doing? You're playing fast and loose; you are playing God." In a sense, the role being played is that of a shaman in society; unfortunately, it is being undercut by our own activities, as well as by the FDA. The American public is being protected from noxious agents by the Food and Drug Administration rules and regulations, which are not drawn to establish priorities. For example, if the prognosis of the patient from the point of view of survival is under two years, the priority relevant to drugs and toxicology and a preclinical workup should certainly be lower than that for an illness in which the prognosis is measured as a normal life expectancy. Supportive agents must be separated from curative agents. Certainly, priority is relevant to those agents that relieve the minor aches and irritations displayed on television commercials for proprietary agents. The priority there has to be different from that for an agent that may conceivably cure, perhaps causing death in 50 percent but cure in 50 percent. In other words, in pharmacology and clinical pharmacology, we have to be given the opportunity relative to those odds from the point of view of triage in life-versus-death situations.

The review committees that interact in advisory fashion with the FDA should be clearly defined in regard to their composition. Membership on these committees should include clinicians who practice medicine—for instance, cardiologists who practice cardiology, not academic people concerned only with preclinical pharmacology. Clinicians know the quality of life and survival and what is essential to their patients.

Consumers should be on the committees. For example, the voluntary societies concerned with cancer or with heart or respiratory disease have a vested interest because they themselves or their family members are suffering from disease, and these laypeople are needed on the committee to interact.

An arbitration system is needed—perhaps one with a federal judgeship, so that the FDA is not both the reviewer and the judge. An alternative individual should be available so that the pharmaceutical industry and those in the special interest groups—like the American Society of Clinical Oncology—can have someone to deal with other than the officials of the FDA. There is always the fear, valid or not, that we could be treated punitively if we confront bureaucracy.

In my own experience, there appears to be a sort of never-never land in administrative jurisdiction. This is particularly evident in the designation of narcotics as being on schedule one or schedule two. For example, I did a study with delta-9-

tetrahydrocannabinol (THC). It took seven different committees one whole year to approve the study. We had joint committees in the FDA, and then the National Institute of Mental Health came into the act. There was also a state committee dealing with narcotics. Finally, it was relayed to the Department of Justice and the narcotics agents. Often they would come by with sidearms and inspect me to make sure that I was not peddling the drugs on the street.

When our program had been cleared, we did an inpatient study, and we were ready to go to our outpatient program when we were told by the FDA that under no circumstances could we give the drug to outpatients, despite the fact that all the protocols had been cleared through numerous committees. Higher officials of the FDA were called to find out why an approved protocol, with $70,000 worth of graduate support—and six psychology graduate students working for me, drawing salary and doing nothing—was not going through. They said, "Dr. Regelson, we know that you can conduct a good study and control your drug, but if we give you permission to go outpatient with this drug, we will have another methadone-type problem on our hands. Every doctor's mother's uncle's cousin will want to do a study, and we won't be able to control it. Therefore, we are not going to allow you to go ahead." The issue had become a social one, not a medical one. However, if one wants to find out if a drug has medicinal value, one does not stop using it because someone may steal a couple of capsules. This will destroy society.

The drug we wanted to work with, THC, is a good prescription drug. We have shown that it has good antianxiety and antidepressive activity for cancer patients. One out of three patients benefited from it. It apparently has a good antiemetic activity. It stimulates appetite and, in cancer patients, it seems to stabilize weight for a period of time.

We have to learn to deal with these social aspects realistically. We have to recognize that all drugs have side effects and that doctors who have prescriptions and narcotics numbers are not peddling pills on the street. So certain drugs should be put into schedule two. I think that heroin is such a drug. In England, heroin has a place in the care of the dying patient. Its addiction problem as related to pain or its effect as a "psychic energizer" indicates that there may be a place for it. Therefore, as a controlled drug it should be available to commissions, because we need as many drugs available to us as we can possibly have. Grof and others (1973) have shown LSD to have value for the dying patient; certainly in the hands of trained therapists it may have a place. Again, as long as it is in schedule one, it is going to be very difficult for us to use a drug of this kind. Society has to say that we cannot be penalized for "abuse" if we have people who are sick. Within the framework of controlled medical environments where people have to be helped, there is no reason why we cannot use them.

In regard to narcotics, I am not a withholder; I am a giver, particularly with cancer patients who suffer pain. We combine them with phenothiazines or haloperidol. We exercise care in using phenothiazines so that we do not wind up with Parkinson patients who are rigid and lose the ability to express themselves because of frozen muscles. Certain drugs clearly can synergize with narcotics to decrease pain.

One of the biggest problems in acute pain is the pain of nerve root discomfort or multiple spinal fractures seen in patients with osteolytic cancer. There is a need for maintenance, so that patients are given a q4H and narcotics on demand under certain circumstances because it takes so long for them to work. There are a buildup in muscle spasm and an increase in pain beyond the threshold for the drug to produce an effect. Nurses and doctors should not be withholding but should consider around-the-clock use of narcotics.

Inhalation anesthesia offers another option. One such agent comes in a handy little sniffer that can be given to the patient. Not every patient can use it. The thing about it is this: patients can learn when the pain is starting to build; they can breathe the drug in; and they can learn to control oblivion if it sets in. Instantly, they are out. Some patients like this and can handle it, yet others are frightened by the sudden loss of consciousness that can accompany it. But patients can learn how to use it. It is relatively safe because the hand drops down when the anesthesia develops. Too frequent use can produce renal tubular injury, but relative to the gain, this may not be considered to be of importance.

In regard to the word *placebo*, I mention a study with normal volunteers in which we attempted to evaluate THC as a potential analgesic. We found that it lowers the pain threshold, so that pain sensitivity is greater. The value of this agent as an analgesic for pain relief is that it relieves anxiety, making it helpful for the despondent patient. To develop this further, we studied 40 out of 40 postoperative cancer patients who were on narcotics. They were five to seven days postoperative and off parenteral intramuscular narcotic. All tubes were out, and they were alimenting. We discovered that every one of these patients was a placebo responder who did not need a narcotic. The placebo effect is a very real one, and we should learn how to use it.

There are numerous intriguing experimental uses of drugs: the role of tryptophane taken orally in enhancing narcotic activity, the place of amino acids in the central nervous system, the use of the phenothiazine tranquilizers, and the use of pentazocine derivatives (except for chronic narcotic users where acute withdrawal symptoms can be a hazard). Some nonnarcotic drugs are actually superior to morphine and, at certain dose levels, are clearly competitive with Demerol and a nonaddicting agent.

In caring for patients, I clearly indicate on charts with orders my feelings about life support. I indicate in writing that I will not use heroic measure and that I will withdraw life support from patients. I so advise the nurses and the house staff. I do not think there should be a living will; I fought legalization of this to the end and stopped it from being passed in Virginia. I am for the individual decision of the physician operating in concert with the family and/or the patient to play a role in this regard, on occasion. However, I do not think there should be legal protection for the withdrawal of life support, because of what happened in Germany. In September 1939, Hitler passed an order legalizing euthanasia for Aryans. By August 1941, about a quarter of a million Germans had been killed.

The bureaucratization of decision making takes away the individual responsibility of the physician. It makes it easy to kill. When we represent an individual in making the final decision, it becomes a moral decision between us and those with whom we interreact. We have to make these decisions openly, but we have to be legally vulnerable, because if we are not, as a physician who knows his colleagues, I know that we can make very serious mistakes. We always have to feel that we are committing murder. It is critical that we have controls on us, and in our society these controls have to be legal ones, making us vulnerable. Do not take vulnerability away from the doctor.

I have strong feelings about autopsy. I used to be as persistent about autopsies as the next person, until I realized after long experience that I learned very little from autopsies unless I was present myself and unless I really wanted the autopsy. I got 100 percent agreement to autopsies by asking for limited autopsies from which only the information I wanted could be gained. For instance, after a patient dies, the family is told the patient had a problem in the chest (which, of course, they know), and it is important to see what happened to that lung cancer as a result of chemotherapy. I ask, "May we go in and look? We will not remove organs; we will just do biopsies as they relate to what is present that we can see. We will be very respectful, and I will be present." If a relationship with the family is developed and indication given that the physician will be there at the autopsy, permission to proceed will be given. On the autopsy consent form, it should be indicated that the doctor is going to be present to find an answer. Otherwise, it cannot be done. The physician's presence hallows the autopsy; otherwise it has no significance.

I believe that we have to have advocates for patients. Nurses and medical personnel all have to play this role. We need holistic approaches. If one is dying or if one's life expectancy is limited, survival must be programmed. Even when dying, one must have something to look forward to the next day, the next week, the next month, because one is not going to die right away. If life is not programmed, if there are no events to look forward to, what is life? A coordinating individual must be available to interact with the family and the patient in a contractual relationship that includes love, attention, and concern. We do not need technicians; we need human beings who care for our patients even through the final moments.

Reference

Grof, S., W. N. Pahnke, L. E. Goodman, and A. A. Kurland. 1973. "Psychedelic Drug Assisted Psychotherapy in Patients with Terminal Cancer. Part Two." In I. K. Goldberg, et al. eds. *Psychopharmacologic Agents for the Terminally Ill and Bereaved*, pp. 91–133. New York: Columbia University Press.

4.
SOME LIMITATIONS OF PSYCHOTROPIC DRUGS IN SUPPORTIVE TREATMENT OF ONCOLOGY PATIENTS

PATRICIA MURRAY

The philosophy underlying our modern pharmacologic and analgesic approach to the management of pain in the cancer patient is probably best summed up by the subtitle of this paper. With this statement, we confront two beliefs of our present health system:

1. It is pills or potents (surgery, radiation, and so forth) that relieve pain and disease.
2. If you have a disease for which we have no pills or potents or in which our pills and potents are ineffective there is nothing more that can be done.

These two beliefs reflect a level of personal awareness and social consciousness that is inadequate and even destructive to the awesome and challenging task of curing and comforting the person with cancer (Cousins 1979).

The major emphasis in management of cancer and treatment and control of its pain is external and institutional. We have invested billions in dollars and more billions in hours of energy and research to alleviate pain and disease through mechanical, technological, and chemical alteration, manipulation, and even disfiguration of the human body. Despite our efforts, cancer and pain persist.

By concentrating our efforts on external approaches to the treatment of disease and pain, we have fostered the belief that healing and health are primarily and almost totally dependent on people and things outside one's personal control. People fully expect that a pill, injection, surgeon's knife, radiation therapy, chemotherapy, and other nostrums will dispense with their disease and pain with little or no effort on their part. Feeling inadequate about their personal recovery powers, people have disassociated from their disease and pain as if these were the province of "official healers" who by a stroke of magic (of whatever form) would make them disappear. As a result, most of us no longer see ourselves as active participants in the healing process.

This expectancy of "other" as powerful and self as impotent is, I suspect, the basis for the ineffectiveness of many of the present protocols used to alleviate pain and disease for cancer patients. Out of impotence grows a resistance, expressed in the body, to protocols meant to relieve pain and disease. Impotence and powerlessness are strong negative emotional sets. Our past response to these powerful negative, internal, emotional experiences of patients has been to manufacture more external and ritualistic approaches to treatment. We build bigger institutions, create larger machines, manufacture more complex and toxic drugs, perform more extensive and disfiguring surgery. We have responded in the way we have learned to handle our own impotence. We have reached out further and higher and placed our potency in external giants that cannot be questioned because they are our main source of power and identity.

Pain and disease hold a meaning, purpose, and experience for each person who is not relieved by our therapeutic modalities. When a person with cancer suffers pain, a question is being raised that does not confine itself to any physiological state. We are geared not to recognize the question marks that pain raises in people. We are not trained to listen to "What is wrong?" "How much longer?" "Why me?" We have been prepared instead to organize the person's pain into a list of complaints that are treatable or untreatable.

In addition, the personal invitation for compassion, understanding, sympathy, honesty, trust, and self-actualization that many of us know how to ask for only through the question mark of pain is bypassed, and the opportunity for the individual to face with support what cannot be faced alone is lost. So also is the opportunity for the person to experience integrity, mastery, and belief in oneself and one's ability to cope with the questions that the pain is raising.

For many patients with cancer and their families the question mark of pain is the reality of death: "Will I die?" "Can I die?" A healing response to pain is a creative response. A creative response to death, to cancer, will involve disruption and recovery. Traditionally, we have concentrated our treatment on the area of physical disruption and recovery. The psychic, social, and spiritual disruption of the person with cancer is often more intense and more painful. And even when there is an attempt to respond to this part of the human person, it is often done in a mechanical and noncreative way.

Our society values anesthesia rather than sensitivity and discipline. Sensitivity is learned through suffering. Sensitivity always implies disruption and recovery or fusion and accommodation. The idea of suffering as a chosen means to the mastery of pain and the control of life and destiny is incomprehensible and shocking to modern medicine and is labeled masochistic. In his book *Medical Nemesis* (in a chapter called "The Killing of Pain"), Ivan Illich states:

> In the capacity for suffering is a possible symptom of health. Suffering is a responsible activity. By equating personal participation in facing unavoidable pain with masochism we justify passive life styles . . . and seek meaning for our passive lives, and power over others by inducing undiagnosable pain and unreliable anxiety such as the hectic life of business executives, the self-punishment of the rat race and intense exposure to violence and sadism on TV and in movies. In such a society advocating new (creative) techniques will inevitably be interpreted as a sick desire for pain [Illich 1976:142].

The position of this paper is that approaches to cancer and pain achieve full effectiveness only when equal attention is given to the meaning and direction pain has for a particular individual. Drugs that alleviate pain will be enhanced when given in conjunction with a therapy that assists the person to face impending disruption and to mobilize energies for active, conscious participation in healing. Disruption—physical, psychological, spiritual—is a normal response to the stress of cancer. A balance is needed that allows patients with cancer to face the disruption and gather together an integrity of self that will mobilize their energies in the direction of healing and health. To assist another person to mobilize energies in the direction of health requires correcting the imbalance in the patient and in our own belief that power lies solely in the potency of the drug or treatment and is not dependent on the patient's inner resources, attitudes, and expectancies (Pelletier 1979).

The work that needs to be done to make our medical management of patients with cancer more effective lies, therefore, as much within ourselves as within our technology. The attitudes and beliefs of the healer will very readily communicate themselves to the patient. Facing one's attitudes and beliefs regarding cancer and pain causes the same disruption in the healer as the experience of serious disease does in the patient. Our attitudes and beliefs are the source of our life energies. If the attitudes and beliefs of healers are characterized by impotence beyond the use of technology, then the healer is limited to technology and not only fails to tap his or her own potency but will also be unable to mobilize or activate the healing powers within patients. Given this situation, the healer is bound to face very limited success, and the constant frustration that such limits produce must be faced (Murray 1981).

To begin to examine our attitudes and beliefs regarding cancer and pain beyond the limits of technology and chemistry involves the possibility of bringing us face to face with our own pessimism, cynicism, and impotence. The pain of this confrontation can never be alleviated by reaching for more powerful technology and more complex chemistry although the temptation to do so will be very strong. For like the patient, we too have been educated in most cases to rely solely and entirely on external powers and protocols. The healer who is willing to bear the discomfort of questioning previous limits and to resist the temptation to find answers in external, mechanical responses opens the self to a broader understanding of the reality of pain and disease. This knowledge and awareness of the total dimensions of pain and disease create the possibility for a more holistic response. In the treatment of cancer, as in no other disease, is this response more challenged. In this disease, both healer and patient experience victimhood when treatment and belief are limited to technology and chemistry. The feelings of impotence and pessimism in both the healer and patient will resist the most powerful treatment protocols (Flach 1974).

An attitude of responsibility for one's own health and a belief that one is a full participant in that process reestablishes the balance of healing power for the patient. The same attitude in the healer not only relieves the healer of the burden of an all-powerful position but also frees the healer to seek more creative alternatives to what has formally been considered incurable disease and intractable pain (Flynn 1980).

What are needed are not only new and better technologies but also a penetrating look into the attitudes and beliefs systems upon which our technologies are founded. If our attitude and belief systems are rooted in impotency, then our technology and chemistry will maintain us all as victims of disease and pain. If our attitude and belief systems are rooted in potency, then we will be masters of our technology, accommodators of our chemistry, and active participants in our own healing.

In summary, the challenge of managing the cancer patient's and the family's pain is as much personal and social as it is medical and psychopharmacological. Modern research in the treatment of pain for cancer for the most part does not reflect the creativity that is born of disruption and recovery. The disruption that needs to take place is a change in the direction of present belief systems that fail to emphasize the ability of the individual to face, with support and understanding, the possibility of death and to find in that confrontation the power to become a participant in the healing of self and a consciously creative human being.

References

Cousins, N. 1979. *The Anatomy of an Illness: Reflections on Healing and Regeneration*. New York: Norton.

Flach, F. 1974. *The Secret Strength of Depression*. New York: Lippincott.

Flynn, P. 1980. *Holistic Health: The Art and Science of Care*. Bowie, Md.: Robert J. Brody Co.

Illich, I. 1976. *Medical Nemesis*. New York: Bantam Books.

Murray, P. 1981. "Nursing Management of the Emotional Components of Pain." In L. B. Marino, ed., *Cancer Nursing*. St. Louis: Mosby.

Pelletier, K. 1979. *Holistic Medicine from Stress to Optimum Health*. New York: Delacorte Press.

5.
PSYCHOLOGICAL HAZARDS OF DRUG THERAPY

Richard S. Blacher

Many undoubtedly would agree on the importance of treating the "whole person" in the management of the dying and bereaved. I should nevertheless like to offer a number of caveats concerning the use of drugs in such cases.

It is difficult to imagine a responsible physician treating a patient in pain without some recourse to analgesic agents, but the very availability of an increased battery of chemical agents poses a danger for the patient. The situations we are discussing are among those that have traditionally demanded of the concerned the greatest sensitivity to the human needs of the patient; they have also caused the doctor a great deal of suffering. Aware of his or her own helplessness in the face of reality, the physician struggles to keep an equilibrium between opposing forces. If one really allows oneself to experience the pain of a dying patient, then one fears being swept up in the emotional turmoil. If one must do this with a number of patients, one may feel absolutely overwhelmed. On the other hand, doctors are concerned lest, in the interest of self-protection, they become insensitive to patients' feelings and present themselves as cold and indifferent. The task becomes one of appreciating the patient's reactions while maintaining one's own balance. In such a situation, the prescription of a tranquilizer may be seductively easy, not as a means of calming the patient but as a substitute for the physician's involvement—as a means of solving one's own dilemma.

Obviously the ideal situation is one in which the drug is given along with the physician's continuing interest and concern.

Another danger is commonly seen when the stark reality of the patient's condition is dealt with by denial on the part of medical attendants and an attempt to minimize reality. It is not at all unusual to find dying patients, in severe pain, undermedicated in many hospitals—probably in most hospitals—and the staff expressing concerns about the patient's becoming addicted to narcotics. This is not a problem of the staff's moral concerns over drug abuse, I believe; colleagues are not so naive as to believe that a patient a few days or weeks from death is a potential addiction problem. Rather, it is an attempt on the part of nurses and doctors to treat the dying patient as curable and thus avoid facing the difficult reality. That patients can be helped to die comfortably and without pain has been amply demonstrated in the hospice program (Saunders 1973). Here an attempt is made to prevent the onset of pain by the frequent administration of analgesic agents in an atmosphere of concern and acceptance of the patient's real situation.

The importance of the presence and impact of the physician on pain and suffering is generally accepted and well documented. Many centuries ago, Hippocrates noted: "Some patients, though conscious that their condition is perilous, recover their health simply through their contentment with the goodness of the physician." The history of medicine since then has been in good measure the history of the placebo, since only in recent years have physicians had many useful drugs available for treating specific conditions (Shapiro 1971). Most treatments in the past have ranged from innocuous to disgusting to downright dangerous. Opium has been used for relief of pain for thousands of years. This, along with cinchona bark for malaria, lime juice for scurvy, and digitalis for heart failure, was the only specific drug available until recently. Nevertheless, physicians have usually been respected members of society and their healing powers have been valued.

Beecher (1955) reviewed the powerful effect of placebo medication on a wide variety of conditions, ranging from headache to angina pectoris to severe postoperative pain. While morphine relieved 75 percent of those with severe postoperative pain, a placebo alone was effective in 35 percent of the cases. This also holds true for cancer patients. The role of the physician is further emphasized in a study by Beecher's anesthesiology group (Egbert et al. 1963). In a carefully monitored evaluation, it was shown that a preoperative visit and discussion of the procedure by the anesthesiologist resulted in a measurable calming effect. This was compared with the use of a preoperative barbiturate, which resulted in patient's coming to the surgical amphitheater drowsy but still anxious.

These studies underline the needs of the patient who is facing death. Medication is, of course, a blessing, but the concerned presence of an understanding physician may fill the real need. Needless to say, medication cannot ease the oft-felt anger of the dying patient. Patients may be angry at themselves for the failure of the body to work right; often the patient is angry at the doctors who have not effected a cure. The anger makes the patient fear abandonment on the part of the physician, and then the patient may become even more angry at this anticipated desertion. The presence of the doctor tends to alleviate the anger. But there is a great temptation for those who tend the patient to slip in and out of the room and write an order for medication instead. While this is understandable on the part of the staff, they cannot expect the patients themselves to be understanding.

For those who are bereaved, there is strong evidence that they, especially spouses are at considerable risk for increased morbidity and mortality (Rees and Lutkins 1967). This is again a situation often calling for the services of an understanding physician. Certainly there may be a need at times for sedation when a survivor is overcome or cannot sleep. Here the danger is twofold. First, a need for much sedation may cover a need to talk about the situation, and drugs may become a substitute for a receptive ear. Second, the working through of grief is a painful but necessary process if the mourner is to be able to continue a productive life. By gratuitously alleviating the painful affects with medication, the physician may contribute to the prevention of the satisfactory resolution of the mourning.

The upwelling of painful and tumultuous feelings in the face of death and bereavement may be especially difficult for members of the medical professions to deal with. First, their main goal is to cure and alleviate suffering and prevent death. Thus, these times are extremely frustrating. Second, the members of the healing professions are chosen on the basis of an ability to be precise. Indeed, only those able to deal with large masses of specific data with exactness are able to get into or pass courses in medical programs. In practice, however, those in the healing arts are faced with enormous areas of ambiguity and imprecision and thus are bound to be in a position of great stress.

In summary, the availability of the physician may be at least as important as the prescription pad in the treatment of the dying and bereaved. The temptation to substitute medication for presence is one we should all struggle against.

> It is the hard lot of the doctor to know that in the end he is always defeated; his victories at best are temporary. Death he can never finally conquer. But death's ally is fear, and this ally the doctor can defeat. Let him help the patient to conquer fear, and he will win many a skirmish; and if he can never hope to win the last grim battle, he can at least do much to rob that ultimate defeat, for his patient and for the patient's family, of the terror that is its most grievous pain [Williams 1975].

References

Beecher, H. K. 1955. "The Powerful Placebo." *Journal of the American Medical Association* (December 24) 159:1602–6.

Egbert, L. D.; A. E. Battit. H. Turndorf, and H. K. Beecher. 1963. "The Value of the Preoperative Visit by an Anesthetist." *Journal of the American Medical Association* (August 17) 185:553–55.

Rees, W. D. and S. G. Lutkins. 1967. "Mortality of Bereavement." *British Medical Journal* (October 7) 4:13–16.

Saunders, C. 1973. "A Death in the Family: A Professional View." *British Medical Journal* (January 6) 1:30–31.

Shapiro, A. K. 1971. "Placebo Effect in Medicine, Psychotherapy, and Psychoanalysis." In A. E. Bergin and S. L. Garfield, eds. *Handbook of Psychotherapy and Behavior Change: Empirical Analysis.* New York: John Wiley and Sons.

Williams, B. A. 1975. "The Greeks Had a Word for It." *New England Journal of Medicine* (October 11) 233.

6.
DRUGS, PHYSICIANS, AND PATIENTS

Irving S. Wright

Physicians and patients have direct concerns in common when dealing with drugs employed in treating multiple diseases—rather than a single disease—in an individual patient particularly in the geriatric patient. The patient may have cancer, and the cancer may be the ultimate and predictable cause of death, but frequently these patients also have heart disease or diabetes or emphysema or any of the many other diseases whose descriptions fill textbooks. As a result, we are confronted also with multiple drug problems. It is not just a matter of prescribing enough sedation or enough analgesia to relieve the patient's pain (although this is of great importance). We are now confronted with the fact that some of these patients are taking so many interacting drugs that the interactions of the drugs may obscure the problems of the disease itself.

A patient of mine returned from Florida with 30 bottles of drugs, all of which had been prescribed for her and all of which she was taking. This patient was extremely ill. She had drifted from one doctor to another, from one specialist to another. We set up the whole army of bottles on my desk. I found that she was taking two kinds of digitalis every day without knowing this, of course, because the names were different and because different doctors had prescribed them. These were enough to produce toxicity and many varieties of symptoms—even death in some patients. She was taking three kinds of diuretics, also without knowing what they were. Sometimes we do prescribe one or two diuretics, but three are usually excessive. This patient had a potassium level of 3.2 mg/%, indicative of a very serious complication of therapy.

This is not only a striking example of overmedication, it is also a very common one. Thus, a problem is created for physicians: they become very protective and defensive, largely because of the long list of possible complications that patients may develop from any particular drug or from the interactions between drugs.

However, lists of complications noted in package inserts, for instance, do not reveal the frequency of their occurrence or whether they are of any importance to the patient. They do indicate that a particular patient may have dizziness, headache, nausea, and so on from taking the drug. The patient can learn this information about side effects from the package inserts, that come with their drugs and he or she may call the doctor and say, "I might die from this drug you have prescribed for me." However, the patient does not know, and even the doctor often does not know, whether the information provided is based on the reported complications' having occurred in only one or two patients (and in some instances it has been with just such infrequency). How can such information be evaluated when half a million people are taking a marketed drug? Maybe there have been others (many? few?) who had similar complications and maybe there were not. Such evidence is not readily available to the doctor. In my opinion, available listings of complications should contain some indication of their relative frequency and severity so that the doctor can evaluate them for their import per se and their relationship to the disease being treated.

These, then, are three of the problems we have—drug interaction, drugs supplied by many different doctors, and the lack of information about what proportion of the patients taking a drug have specific side effects. Patients should not panic when they see the long list of possible complications that have been reported from many cases. These are sensitive and controversial areas that remain to be considered at greater length so that they may be resolved more satisfactorily. Any group or commission that is charged with dealing with the care of the elderly, even into the death period, should review these problems very carefully, for they affect the care given our patients today.

As a patient nears death, it is sometimes difficult to determine how many or which of the apparent symptoms are due to impending death and how many or which are due to the medication being prescribed. I have seen several patients who appear to be comatose and on whom all had about given up. Then it was found that they had been receiving four or five different kinds of analgesics and sedatives whose cumulative effects were very striking. When taken off all drugs, or perhaps kept on a mild one, the patient regained consciousness and the ability to function in a satisfactory fashion. Obviously, the patient was not as near the end as the caregivers had thought.

As we are able to reach solutions for such problems, no doubt we will be creating other problems to be solved. In the course of time, we must strive to better separate and sort one problem from another.

7
PROBLEMS OF POLYPHARMACY

David M. Benjamin

The use of more than one drug in a patient constitutes polypharmacy. Numerous epidemiologic studies have reported that the probability of occurrence of an adverse drug reaction was directly related to the number of drugs a patient received and the duration of administration. While individual variations in response to therapy may serve as a partial explanation for the large number of adverse drug reactions encountered, today's literature is replete with reports of a second, presumably unrelated drug's altering a patient's response to a previously well-tolerated medication.

Because it is common for patients with chronic malignant diseases to be treated with many medications concomitantly, this population of patients is particularly likely to experience some sort of adverse drug effect. Moreover, the fact that several physicians may be involved in the overall care of a patient further compounds the problem, since Dr. A (an oncologist, for example) may have no knowledge of medications prescribed by Dr. B (a psychiatrist, perhaps). If the patient also has additional underlying medical problems such as diabetes, epilepsy, or asthma, then the probability of disposing this patient toward greater morbidity by precipitating adverse drug reactions is even further increased.

It is difficult, if not impossible, to avoid polypharmacy in many patients. However, if readers are familiar with the various types of pharmacokinetic drug interactions that can occur and the underlying mechanisms involved in precipitating drug interactions, they should be able to prescribe drugs more judiciously and thus provide better patient care and precipitate a lower incidence of iatrogenic adverse drug interactions.

Basically, pharmacokinetic drug interactions can be divided into four categories: drugs affecting the (1) absorption, (2) distribution, (3) metabolism, and (4) excretion of a second drug. However, it is also possible for two drugs with similar pharmacodynamic activities to have an additive effect upon one another and thus enhance side effects common to both agents (e.g., phenobarbital and phenytoin administered concurrently, in therapeutic doses, may precipitate sedation, ataxia, or nystagmus). Other drug interactions can involve two drugs with different pharmacologic effects that interact through a common pathway or site of action. For example, tricyclic antidepressants, which block the reuptake of norepinephrine into the adrenergic neuron, may also block the uptake of certain adrenergic neuron blocking agents, such as guanethidine, which is used in the treatment of hypertension. Therefore, hypertensive patients whose blood pressure is well controlled while receiving guanethidine alone, may become hypertensive when a tricyclic agent such as imipramine or amitriptyline is added to their regimen.

Pharmacokinetic Factors Affecting Absorption

Absorption of drugs from the gastrointestinal tract is dependent upon many factors, including gut motility, volume and pH of secretions, presence or absence of food, regional blood flow, drug formulation (tablet disintegration and solute dissolution rates), and aqueous and lipid solubility. Anticholinergic agents and antacids containing Al^{+3} reduce peristalsis, prolong gastric emptying time, retard the rates of tablet disintegration and dissolution and thus interfere with normal drug absorption. Other agents promoting hypermotility (e.g., cathartics) may decrease the absorption of drug formulations with slow disintegration rates, such as enteric-coated or time-released preparations.

Drug absorption from the gastrointestinal tract is generally considered to be best typified by simple diffusion across a lipoid membrane with water-filled pores. On the basis of this assumption, these membranes are most permeable to the nonionized lipid-soluble forms of drugs. Since many drugs are either weak acids or bases, the passage of these drugs across membranes becomes a function of the ambient pH and the pKa of the drug as related in the Henderson-Hasselbalch equations.

For an acid:
$$pKa = pH + \log \frac{\text{Molecular concentration of unionized acid}}{\text{Molecular concentration of ionized acid}}$$

For a base:
$$pKa = pH + \log \frac{\text{Molecular concentration of ionized base}}{\text{Molecular concentration of unionized base}}$$

Since the administration of alkalizing agents ($NaHCO_3$) or agents that promote HCl secretion (caffeine, alcohol) affect gastric pH, it is quite reasonable to assume that the absorption of drugs susceptible to this effect would be altered.

In addition to an effect on pH, alkalizing agents also have an effect on drug solubility. Since only drugs that have become dissolved in gastric or intestinal fluid are available for absorption, the delicate balance between the degree of ionization and solubility must also be considered. A perfect example of this relationship can be seen with aspirin. Aspirin (acetylsalicylic acid) is a weak acid with a pKa of 3.5. Therefore, using the Henderson-Hasselbalch equation for weak acids and assuming a gastric pH in the range of 1–2, we can determine that of the aspirin in solution, the predominant species is the unionized, absorbable form. However, the total amount of aspirin available for absorption would be the product of the concentration in solution and the percentage of aspirin in the unionized form. Although concomitant administration of $NaHCO_3$ or other alkalinizing agents would decrease the percentage of aspirin present in the unionized form, it also increases the aqueous solubility of aspirin and thereby increases the rate of absorption. In this instance, the effect of $NaHCO_3$ on aspirin absorption is chiefly an effect on aspirin solubility rather than on displacing the equilibrium between ionized and unionized form to increase the concentration of unionized drug present.

Additional factors influencing the absorption of drugs from the gastrointestinal tract involve the presence or absence of food in the stomach (penicillin G versus penicillin V) and the formation of insoluble complexes due to the presence of sequestering or chelating agents (e.g., bivalent cations form insoluble complexes with tetracyclines, and cholestyramine binds acidic drugs like warfarin and thus reduces drug absorption).

Pharmacokinetic Factors Affecting Drug Distribution

The distribution of drugs to their sites of action, metabolism, and excretion occurs chiefly through transport in blood plasma. As drugs enter the plasma, a percentage of the molecules in solution generally become associated with (bound to) one of the plasma proteins. Most drugs are bound primarily to albumin, but alpha and beta globulins are also involved with the transport of some drugs.

The bond between drug molecule and transport protein may be weak or strong; it may be strictly an ionic bond based on a charged molecule's attraction for an oppositely charged region of a protein, or it may involve hydrophobic or hydrogen bonds. In any event, an equilibrium is established in plasma between bound drug and free drug. Since only unbound drug is available to interact with the appropriate receptor, the amount of drug bound to protein and the strength of the bond are major determinants in the expression of pharmacologic activity.

Certain groups of drugs (e.g., organic acids) or classes of compounds appear to share a limited number of binding sites on protein molecules. Although some of the members of this group of drugs may attach to the same protein-binding sites, the strength of the bond (affinity) will differ among the individual drug molecules themselves. Drugs with the greatest affinity for the binding sites are held to protein by the strongest bonds and will also displace drug molecules with lesser affinities from their binding sites.

A classical example of two drugs competing for the same protein-binding site is the interaction between phenylbutazone and coumarin anticoagulants. Coumarin anticoagulants (e.g., warfarin) are approximately 98 percent bound to plasma proteins at physiologic concentrations. Therefore, anticoagulant activity is produced by the 2 percent of the drug that remains free in plasma. Concomitant administration of phenylbutazone, a pyrazoline-type nonsteroidal antiinflammatory agent that is also 98 percent bound to plasma proteins, causes phenylbutazone to compete for protein-binding sites already occupied by warfarin. The result is that some warfarin is displaced from its binding sites, causing the concentration of free warfarin to increase. This increase leads to an enhanced anticoagulant effect, which is usually recognized clinically by purpura, hematuria, and an exaggerated increase in the prothrombin time.

Because coumarins are 98 percent bound and 2 percent free, minimal displacement of these compounds from their binding sites causes large changes in pharmacologic response. An increase of only 1 percent in the amount of free drug circulating in plasma is tantamount to increasing the activity of the drug 1½ times (from 2 to 3 percent free drug). Therefore, highly bound drugs that exert their pharmacologic effects through low free drug concentrations have a greater potential to produce potentiated responses when displaced from binding sites than drugs do that are bound to a lesser degree.

The concept that drugs exert their pharmacologic effects in proportion to their free drug concentrations is axiomatic. Therefore any clinical situation that alters the ratio of bound to free drug is likely to produce a corresponding change in the expression of that drug's pharmacologic activity. Increases in free drug concentration produce enhanced or potentiated activity, while decreases in free drug concentration produce attenuated responses.

The major factor contributing to alterations in the ratio of free to bound drug is plasma protein concentration. Patients suffering from chronic debilitating diseases may have an impaired ability to synthesize albumin in the liver or may lose large amounts of protein in their urine. Impaired hepatic synthesis of albumin and marked proteinuria both have the effect of reducing the number of binding sites available to sequester the drug and thus, in effect, increasing the concentration of free drug. When hypoalbuminemia is recognized in a patient, great care should be taken to administer the smallest possible dose of a drug (especially a highly bound drug) until the clinical response can be observed. Gradual titration toward a desired therapeutic response will decrease the likelihood of saturating all the protein-binding sites and thus producing a greater than expected response as a result of an increased circulating concentration of free drug. Moreover, patients with chronic renal failure may produce plasma proteins that have an abnormally low capacity to bind certain drugs (e.g., phenytoin) and thus predispose them to enhanced responsiveness and an increased susceptibility to toxicity.

Pharmacokinetic Factors Affecting Drug Metabolism

The magnitude of effect and the duration of action of many drugs are directly related to the rate at which a compound is biotransformed (metabolized) to a new chemical entity. This new chemical entity derived from the parent (original) drug molecule is called a metabolite. In general, metabolites are usually less active than the parent compound (although some drugs must be activated by a metabolic step), and for this reason metabolism is sometimes referred to as detoxification.

Although biotransformation may lead to a metabolite that is either more active or less active than the parent compound, metabolites in general are more water-soluble than the corresponding parent compounds from which they were derived. Increasing the aqueous solubility of a compound decreases the amount of reabsorption that can occur in the kidney and promotes the compound's elimination (excretion) from the body.

Most drugs are metabolized by the microsomal enzymes of the liver. These enzymes are located in the smooth endoplasmic reticulum of the hepatocyte and require molecular oxygen,

NADPH, and cytochrome P-450 to metabolize the substrate.

The chemical reactions that take place during drug metabolism can be divided into two classes: nonsynthetic and synthetic. The nonsynthetic reactions usually involve oxidation, reduction, or hydrolysis of the parent compound and frequently generate a compound with a reactive group (e.g., -OH, or -NH$_2$). This reactive intermediate can form a more polar derivative when coupled with glucuronic acid, an ethereal sulfate, an amino acid, or an acetyl donor during a synthetic (or conjugation) reaction. Pharmacokinetic drug interactions involving the metabolism of a drug arise when the activity of the enzymes catalyzing either the synthetic or nonsynthetic reactions are altered by previous or concurrent administration of an agent that modifies the capacity of certain enzymes to metabolize substrate. Depending on the nature of the modifying agent, metabolism may be enhanced (enzyme induction) or inhibited.

The classical enhancing agent is phenobarbital. Phenobarbital induces the formation of new enzymatic protein in the smooth endoplasmic reticulum of the hepatocyte, causing drugs that are substrates for these enzymes to be metabolized at a greater rate and to have a shorter plasma half-life. Drugs that are metabolized by the same enzyme system may compete with one another for the active site on a limited amount of enzyme. This competitive antagonism may be a significant mechanism by which one drug inhibits the rate of metabolism of a second drug.

Hundreds of drugs, insecticides, gases, carcinogens, and other chemicals have been shown to induce microsomal enzyme activity. However, the characteristic pharmacologic actions of these compounds are quite different, and there is no apparent relationship between their actions or structures and their capacity as inducers. The only similarity among these compounds is that most inducers are very lipid-soluble at physiological pH. Some of the more common classes of drugs known to induce microsomal enzyme activity are barbiturates, anticonvulsants, sulfonylureas, antihistamines, and phenothiazines.

Another phenomenon associated with enhanced drug metabolism, yet differing from enzyme induction, is commonly known as "the first-pass effect." Because drugs absorbed from the gastrointestinal tract (with the exception of the lower rectum) enter the liver via the portal circulation before entering the general circulation, any drug that is extensively cleared from the plasma by the liver will have a lower systemic availability than one might expect. Since this enhanced hepatic clearance usually occurs with the first dose of drug—the first time that drug passes through the liver—the phenomenon has been named the first-pass effect. Subsequently, the extraction mechanism becomes saturated with drug and hepatic clearance decreases. Under steady-state conditions (repeated daily administration of a set dose of medication), the first-pass effect needs to be considered only: (1) during the administration of the first dose and (2) following discontinuation of the multiple dosing regimen and subsequent renewal of drug therapy.

Not all drugs are subject to a first-pass effect. Several of the more important drugs known to be involved in this phenomenon are propranalol, lidocaine, and propoxyphene. Unfortunately, there is no way to predict whether or not a drug will be subject to this effect. However, a diminished clinical effect in response to what is believed to be a therapeutic dose of medication should alert the prescribing physician to the possibility of an abnormal disposition of the drug.

Pharmacokinetic Factors Affecting Drug Excretion

Renal excretion of drugs is related to a variety of physiologic and pharmacokinetic factors. Although charged, water-soluble metabolites are excellent candidates for excretion, physiologic parameters such as heart rate, cardiac output, peripheral resistance, and urinary pH all play important roles in modifying the concentration of metabolite present in tubular urine and the rate at which plasma enters the renal system to initiate the first step in urine formation.

Assuming an absence of pathological factors that might impair normal hemodynamics or cause frank renal failure, the renal excretion of drugs is chiefly a function of the concentration and molecular charge of a drug molecule or metabolite. The more polar a metabolite, the greater the chances that it will pass through the glomerulus and become part of the tubular urine. Metabolites that are more lipid-soluble can be reabsorbed into the systemic circulation and thus decrease the efficiency of the excretion process. Other drugs (e.g., penicillin) are actively secreted into tubular urine and thus cause their rate of excretion to be greater than expected.

Many drugs are known to affect the pH of tubular urine. When these agents are administered before or concurrently with a second agent whose pKa lies within a range susceptible to changes in pH (7.5–10.5 for bases; 3.0–7.5 for acids), the ratio of the amount of drug being reabsorbed to the amount of drug being excreted can be significantly affected. A primary example of the use of this phenomenon to aid patients is in the case of phenobarbital toxicity. Phenobarbital, unlike most of the other barbiturates, has a low pKa, near 7.2. Administration of $NaHCO_3$ to the phenobarbital-intoxicated patient promotes the conversion of the molecule to its ionized form and thus increases the rate of renal excretion and elimination from the body. Similarly, administration of the acidifying agent NH_4Cl converts many amphetamine-like drugs to more ionized species and thus increases the efficiency of the kidneys in ridding the body of these dangerous drugs.

In addition to passive reabsorption, the kidney has several active or carrier-medicated transport systems for handling the reabsorption and secretion of many organic acids and bases. Since there are a limited number of receptor sites available for occupation, it is possible for one drug to compete with another for "available space." Penicillins are an excellent example of a class of agents that are actively secreted into tubular urine by a specific transport mechanism. With typical administration of penicillin G, the half-life in the human organism is on the order of 30 minutes. Prior treatment of an individual with the drug probenecid (a drug that is also secreted by the same transport system that handles penicillin) competes for receptor sites and thus causes less penicillin to be secreted and the plasma half-life to be extended to several hours in man.

Although the kidney is the organ chiefly responsible for drug excretion, other, less important routes also function to facilitate drug excretion in man. Excretion of drugs into the bile followed by elimination in the feces is a pathway of secondary importance, especially in patients with compromised renal function. Knowledge of a drug's extrarenal excretion pattern may be an important factor in selecting among several drugs that might conceivably be prescribed for an older patient or a patient with decreased renal function. For example, although all tetracyclines possess the same spectrum of antibacterial activity, chlortetracycline is more dependent on biliary excretion for its elimination than the other tetracyclines are. Therefore, this would be the tetracycline of choice for a patient with compromised renal function.

In addition to biliary excretion, other secondary routes of excretion include the tears, saliva, expired air, and milk. Of these, expired air is of importance mainly for the elimination of anesthetic gases and vapors, while excretion of drugs in the milk of nursing mothers is a very real route for administering drugs (sometimes inadvertently) to neonates. Although not of significance in the overall elimination of a drug from the body, salivary drug levels represent a new means of estimating blood drug levels. Correlations between salivary and plasma levels of digoxin and theophylline have already been established, and current trends indicate that salivary drug levels may represent a highly accessible body fluid that can be obtained by noninvasive techniques to monitor plasma drug concentrations.

Predicting Adverse Drug Interactions

Although there is no known way to definitely predict when an adverse drug interaction will occur, there are some steps that physicians can take to lessen the likelihood of such reactions.

1. Obtain a complete history of all drugs currently being taken by the patient before prescribing an additional medication. This includes vitamins, laxatives, aspirin, and any other over-the-counter drugs used for allergy, colds, and occasional aches and pains.

2. Be acquainted with the basic pharmacology of all concomitant medications. From a pharmacology text determine the following:

a. chemical class—organic acid, organic base, phenothiazine, thiazide

b. pharmacologic activity—analgesic, diuretic, monoamine oxidase inhibitor

c. common side effects and pathways of expression—dry mouth and tachycardia due to anticholinergic effect.

d. basic ADME information—(ADME stands for absorption, distribution, metabolism, and excretion); basic information should include (1) the site and extent of absorption; (2) the extent of binding to plasma proteins; (3) the half-life (T½) of the drug, as well as the major metabolic pathways and principal metabolites; and (4) the major pathway of excretion.

3. Become familiar with the blood or plasma levels associated with therapeutic and toxic responses. Try to learn the differences between ng/ml (1 nanogram = 10^{-9} grams or 10^{-3} micrograms), μ/ml (1 microgram = 10^{-6} grams or 10^{-3} milligrams) and mg% (also known as mg/dl or mg/100 ml = 10μ/ml).

4. If affiliated with a medical center offering certain blood-level determinations, talk with the head of the laboratory, who can give important details on when to obtain blood samples (in relation to the time of administration of the previous dose of drug). At steady-state (the time when the amount of drug entering the body each day equals the amount excreted), blood-level determinations can give an index of the lowest (trough) level of the drug by means of a blood sample taken just before administration of the next dose. Peak blood levels (following oral administration) are generally achieved 1 to 3 hours following the administration of an oral dose except when the drug under evaluation has an exceptionally long absorptive phase (e.g., digoxin). As a rule of thumb, steady-state is usually reached after a minimum of 6 half-lives' time. Therefore, drugs with short half-lives reach steady-state before drugs with longer half-lives.

5. Consider the pathophysiological state of the patient. Liver disease can produce hypoalbuminemia, which leads to a decrease in plasma protein binding and/or impaired metabolism, which is accompanied by an increase in the half-life of many drugs. Renal disease can impair the excretion of drugs and thus increase the half-life of the compound (e.g., digoxin and gentamicin).

6. Evaluate the information compiled on these drugs in terms of the effects each drug might have on the absorption, distribution, me-

tabolism, and excretion of other concomitant medications. Bear in mind that drugs of the same chemical class and blood-level concentrations are more likely to interact than drugs with dissimilar properties.

For a more in-depth discussion of pharmacokinetics and drug interactions, see the references.

References

Benet, L. Z., ed. 1976. "The Effect of Disease States on Drug Pharmacokinetics." *American Pharmacology Association/Academy of Pharmacological Science*.
Levy, G., ed. 1974. *Clinical Pharmacokinetics*. American Pharmacological Association.
Morelli, H. F. and K. L. Melmon. 1968. "The Clinician's Approach to Drug Interactions." *California Medicine* 109:380–89.
Prescott, L. F. 1969. "Pharmacokinetic Drug Interactions." *Lancet* 2:1239–43.
Robinson, D. S. 1975. "Pharmacokinetic Mechanisms of Drug Interactions." *Postgraduate Medicine* 57:55–62.

8.
SUICIDE BY DRUG OVERDOSE

Bruce L. Danto

Introduction

At no other time in the history of this and most other countries have there been more people using medications that, when taken in large quantities, can result in death. Since the introduction of tranquilizers, barbiturates, and nonbarbiturate hypnotic agents, those who attempt and commit suicide have a veritable arsenal of potentially lethal agents from which to choose in order to arrange their exit from the planet Earth.

Common Drugs of Overdose and Their Medical Management

The major tranquilizers with the highest milligram potency and lowest dosage have the fewest reported deaths from overdose ingestions. The pharmacologic effects of these drugs cause the physician to use some caution. These drugs delay gastric emptying, and for this reason, overdose can be treated with lavage. Because they exert an antiemetic effect, antiemetic agents are of no benefit. Because they lower the convulsive seizure threshold, stimulant drugs should be used with extreme caution, for they might produce seizures. Phenothiazines reverse the effect of epinephrine and should not be used to support the cardiovascular system. Preferred for that purpose would be levarterenol. Dialysis should be avoided in treatment, for these drugs are quickly bound to nondialyzable proteins.

The minor tranquilizers pose problems in terms of lethality. Ingesting one month's supply of meprobamate, for example, would result in death. Although dialysis would work for this particular drug, it would not work for an overdose of chlordiazepoxide or the other minor tranquilizers in that some are dialyzable. They too can be highly lethal when ingested in large amounts and have greater lethality than the major tranquilizers.

Among the antidepressant medications, there are two basic types, the tricyclics and the monoamine oxidase inhibitors. Each type of antidepressant carries the same lethality potential, and a two weeks' supply could be fatal when ingested at one time. Additional serious problems arise with the monoamine oxidase inhibitors. They are very toxic when combined with other drugs, particularly the tricyclics, and when combined with foodstuffs containing tryamine, such as cheese.

Treatment of overdose by these tricyclics involves efforts to relieve their strong anticholinergic action. If the drug is combined with anti-Parkinson agents, bladder and bowel paralysis or cardiac dysrhythmias may occur. Dialysis is without value for these drugs but is effective when used early for the treatment of monoamine oxidase inhibitors overdose.

Treatment of overdose by barbiturates is relatively uncomplicated. In the majority of cases, simple medical supportive care is all that is needed (Davis 1973). The latter concept involves conscientious nursing care, keeping the airway clear, rehydration, temperature control, management of hypotension and renal function, and possible alkinization by combining intravenous sodium bicarbonate with intravenous glucose and water if the drug ingested is phenobarbital. With the nonbarbiturate, glutehimide, the lethal dose is only 10 times the usual nightly dose. Its clinical picture is similar to that of barbiturate toxicity but there are peripheral cholinergic signs as well, e.g., gastrointestinal paralysis, dilated pupils, laryngospasm, and apnea. Coma, when present, is longer than for the corresponding dose of barbiturates. In instances of overdosage for either of the latter two drugs, current practice excludes the use of analeptic drugs.

With barbiturates and nonbarbiturate hypnotics, deaths have been reported. The development of life-sustaining techniques and intensive care units in general hospitals has markedly reduced the number of suicides that would have occurred if such service had not been available. Advanced technology in the areas of communication and emergency medical transportation has also helped to reduce the number of fatalities.

However, one should not be fooled by such drugs as being the only ones about which concern should be expressed in the case of a patient who has overdosed. Donlon and Tupin (1977) studied five cases of deaths due to overdose of thioridazine and mesoridazine. Both drugs resemble tricyclic drugs in that they can be lethal because of cardiac effects due to cardiotoxicity. They psychiatrist in particular must be mindful of this possibility, especially if treating a suicidal schizophrenic person.

Of no less importance are analgesic agents such as aspirin and propoxyphene napsylate, which are prescribed in even greater numbers for all kinds of pain control problems. Obviously, in the case of aspirin use, the amount is greater because it is available as an over-the-counter preparation and the consumer self-prescribes it. Warren et al. (1974) reported on a case of proporyphenenapsylate overdose where the patient could not be revived, owing to early cardiorespiratory arrest. Dialysis, gastric absorption by activated charcoal, the recommended treatment modalities for this type of toxicity, and the employment of naloxone hydrochloride were totally unsuccessful in treating this case. Although the blood level of that agent in the 19-year-old subject was 0.5 to 0.8 gm, the case was further complicated by his having also ingested large quantities of aspirin.

Other combinations of drugs have been shown to have more lethal consequences than when only one drug is taken in overdose. Rada et al. (1975) reported two cases of an overdose of chlordiazepoxide and alcohol and pointed out that before their report, most physicians considered the minor tranquilizer involved to be totally safe and nonproductive of death when taken in overdose. The blood plasma of one patient in their study contained 2 mcg/ml of chlordiazepoxide and 0.35 percent of alcohol. In their second case, the plasma level of chlordiazepoxide was 7.7 mcg/ml and of alcohol, 0.19 percent. The ominous note from these case reports stems from the fact that this minor tranquilizer is often used in the treatment of alcoholism. Because alcoholic persons in treatment frequently slip and resume drinking, these cases should suggest that the physician treating such a patient refrain from prescribing large amounts, assess the depression and suicidal potential in the patient, and caution the patient about drinking and using the minor tranquilizers in combination.

Drug Automatism and Barbiturate Overdose Suicide

According to Dorpat, (1974) many physicians claim that some fatal and nonfatal cases of barbiturate poisoning are caused by drug automatism and therefore are really accidental. The ingestion of a therapeutic dose of barbiturate causes the person to lose track of taking the drug and therefore, to keep repeating the dose until lapsing into unconsciousness.

Dorpat argues that if a patient were to take a sleeping pill every 15–20 minutes, after three or four tablets the patient would fall asleep. Since the fatal dose of barbiturates is 10–20 times the hypnotic dose, it would be impossible for the patient to die from drug automatism, based on a gradual increase of an excessive amount of such drugs. Furthermore, at autopsy in lethal overdose cases involving barbiturates frequently such large concentrations of drugs are found in the tissues that it is implied that there must have been a single, large ingestion of the drug—many pills at one time, not one pill at a time over a long period of time.

Hard-Core Addiction and Drug Ingestion Suicide

It is important to understand that there is no homogeneous group of hard-core addicts. Many youths who are turned on to drugs may differ from those who use drugs as a way of life. Use of one type of drug may vary from one group to another. Racial, situational, cultural, and socioeconomic factors have been postulated and studied. Among the most important factors is that of the psychology behind reaching out for and continuing to use drugs in a risk-taking fashion.

Frederick et al. (1973) stated that most addicts are aware that they place their lives in jeopardy by using drugs. They hear about mainline deaths of friends and others who make up this fringe group. The word about bad and lethal trips always gets out.

Frederick states further that the death rate from drug addiction populations has been extremely high; the nonnatural death rate for addicts is five times greater than for the general population, and accidental deaths among addicts are twice as high. In keeping with this self-destructive life-style, or better yet, death style of the addict population, O'Donnell (1964) found that addicts have a higher rate of suicide than the general population.

Frosch et al. (1967) found that one-fifth of 34 patients who had ingested LSD experienced feelings of depression, hopelessness, and some suicidal ideation. Pierce (1967) found a higher than average suicide rate among addicts he studied in England.

Frederick et al. (1973) conducted a study using the Zung Depression Scale with a group of 78 hard-core addicts admitted three months earlier to a methadone maintenance program. Another 20 hard-core addicts who had not been on methadone were also tested. Various control groups were compared, e.g., 50 delinquents who had records but without drug abuse and 30 normals chosen also for comparison. In all groups, the males predominated at about 70 percent; their ages ranged from 15 to 26, and the group was one-third Protestant, one-third Jewish, and one-third nonchurchgoers.

Results of this study revealed a higher tendency toward depression among the drug users who were on methadone; their scores were 60 or more. In the drug addiction groups, less than half scored in the normal range on the Depression Scale, but in the control groups, two-thirds scored in the normal range. Finally, this study revealed that suicide attempts within these groups of whites were higher among the addicts than among nonaddicts, compared with a general white population. An empirical view heard by the researchers was that traits of depression and suicide were present after the onset of addiction and during abstinence following addiction.

Psychodynamics of Oral Ingestion Suicidal Behavior

Most persons who use medication as a method for suicide are frightened of pain and violence. They want a quiet exit, one that is like sleep. In Freudian terms, this would represent an oral type of coping behavior. It would also be consistent with a more passive-dependent personality style, reflecting a passive-dependent type surrender to the pressures associated with the development of hopelessness and loss of self-esteem. The ingester thinks, "Now I have these problems off my back. I can rest easy. I can go to sleep and make all the problems disappear. I can end the pain. I'm not resentful or enraged by anything in life. I just want out. I want a peaceful end to suffering. I just know I don't have a future. Everything I have tried has failed."

For this person there are no fantasies of wanting survivors to remember the painful image of a gunshot wound or some other fatal mutilating injury. There is nothing exhibitionistic about this mode of death compared with bridge jumpers, skyjackers, assassins, and snipers. One dies as one has lived, mainly unnoticed and quietly. The death is almost an apology for troubling anyone. The pills have blocked out and sedated away all concern about or interest in the effects of the death on survivors. All the suicide can see is the end to pain and suffering; the pills offer a painless way to go.

Suicide Prevention for Drug Ingesters

Aside from the formidable addict population, there is a vast number of potential drug overdosers in this country. According to a 1978 *FDA Drug Bulletin,* despite some declining trends in the use of sedative hypnotics in recent years, they are still the most prescribed medications in the world. In 1976, in the United States, 128 million prescriptions for this type of drug were filled. Hypnotic agents alone accounted for 27 million prescriptions. These numbers make suicide prevention almost impossible.

The general fields of medicine known to write the most prescriptions for these drugs are family/general practice, internal medicine, and neurology/psychiatry. Physicians in these fields write the greatest number of outpatient prescriptions. The logical place to implement a suicide prevention program is with physicians who prescribe these drugs with almost reckless abandon.

Murphy (1972) conducted a suicide study in St. Louis, Missouri. He found that in about 50 percent of the cases, the suicided patient had seen a physician within six months of death. This fact, coupled with the high number of hypnotic and tranquilizer prescriptions written by physicians, should call for emergency measures and wise policies that insist upon a restrictive policy regarding the issuance of such prescriptions. Furthermore, it should be viewed as just plain good medical procedure to inquire of patients why they cannot sleep, why they have lost their appetite, what they think about when nervous or depressed, and what major events are happening in their life. It should also be a matter of routine to inquire about sex drive, ability to work, how difficult it is to arise in the morning, hobbies or interests, and how well the patient is getting along with others. A physician should be able to recognize qualities of sadness or lifelessness in a patient. The physician should not be afraid to ask about thoughts of suicide or about experiences with suicide attempts. The physician should inquire about accidents, driving habits, and numbers and types of traffic offenses and should ask a depressed person about firearms and medications kept in the home.

Having determined that the person is depressed, the physician should not prescribe an amount of medication that would last more than a week. The physician should see this patient at least once a week to get to know him or her and to convey to the patient the physician's interest and solicitude. A prescription for large amounts of tranquilizers or hypnotic agents is more than a suggestion to the patient to end it all or take a big sleep so that the doctor can be left alone in peace.

This advice does not appear to be radical. After all, the average physician would not hesitate to have a patient return often for a check on anticoagulant or digitalis medication to guard against a hazardous degree of titer or one that would induce an adverse reaction. This advice is consistent with that experience.

The difference here lies in the fact that the doctor must recognize the lethality and potential adverse reactions of prescribed sedatives and tranquilizers.

There are other measures for prevention of suicide open to the physician. One is prescribing a medication that has a sedative effect but that does not have the potentially lethal effect, even when taken in overdose. Most antihistaminic preparations fall into this category of agents. Reading before retiring for the night and taking a warm bath might also help the patient with sleep problems to relax. Having the patient call the doctor on a "rap line" at night to discuss some feelings or events of the day might help. The latter measure also has the advantage of reducing the isolation felt by a patient who lives alone.

Benzodiazepines can be used, but caution must be exercised. It was noted previously that when these are taken in overdose or in combination with large amounts of alcohol, the results can be fatal. Certainly, small prescriptions for them would protect the depressed patient from a lethal overdose reaction better than an overdose from a barbiturate or a nonbarbiturate hypnotic overdose.

The physician who feels trapped by a patient who has overdosed with either a large prescription the physician has written or a large cache of pills the patient has accumulated for suicide must exercise care and control over feelings. It is human for any physician to resent being "had" or manipualted by such a patient. Resentment can be expressed in terms of feeling the patient was not fair, of feeling disappointed and concerned about the patient's almost losing life or acting to take it. However, the physician needs to continue seeing the patient and may want to seek a concomitant psychiatric consultation to offer more specific help than a prescription can offer. It also helps if the physician contacts the family, with the patient's permission, for it may be necessary to offer support to the patient through the family. Also, if the family has large amounts of medication in the home, these should be kept locked.

Finally, the physician should have an opportunity to assess whether the family really wants the patient who overdoses to end up alive. Perhaps some member or members have been unconsciously encouraging suicide as a solution to their own feelings or problems.

Nursing and emergency room personnel can play an important role in the care of the suicide attempter who has overdosed. The person should be greeted with comments like, "I'm glad you're alive. We're happy to have you here. That's what a hospital is for. You must have been pretty upset. I hope we can help you find a way of coping with your unhappiness."

All too often what really happens is that the patient is unceremoniously brought in by the police, who wryly state in loud voices, "Another psycho is here who attempted suicide with an overdose." The embarrassed patient, if conscious, is then taken into a room, undressed, gowned, and placed on a cart where the word "psycho" is scrawled on the sheet for everyone to see.

Frequently, patients who are initiated into hospital staff anger in this manner soon make another attempt at suicide. In an unpublished study I conducted of all hospital emergency rooms in Wayne County, Michigan, from 1970 to 1972, I was shocked to learn that in 70 percent of suicide attempter cases of all methods, the disposition was unknown. That meant the patients had walked out. In turn, it meant that the attempters/patients felt that no one cared, that they were viewed as being lepers, and the world in general was telling them to find another bottle of pills.

For persons who overdose or attempt suicide by any method, it is imperative that follow-up care be offered. This may be in the form of psychiatric or psychological treatment. It may be in the form of an interested doctor calling them at home later to check on them and let them know the physician cares. Similarly, the suicide prevention or crisis intervention agency, which may have intervened once the attempt was either threatened or made, should contact the patients after hospital emergency care to let them know that the agency has human concern for people who call asking for help.

This paper has focused on the incidence of overdose suicide and attempted suicide. It has summarized common drugs used, the kinds of adverse reactions encountered, and the types of medical methods to be used in treating the overdoses.

Negated as a factor in drug overdose was the belief in drug automatism. A relationship between drug addiction and suicide was discussed in terms of recent studies about depression among addicts. Some psychodynamic concepts about ending frustration and tension, as well as seeing sleep as a pleasant form of death, were discussed as possibilities. Specific points about what can be done by using crisis intervention and suicide prevention were discussed in terms of clinical practice at the hospital emergency room, doctor's office, and crisis center.

It should be apparent that working with the suicide attempter who ingests drugs requires active intervention, therapeutic commitment to the patient, contact with the family when possible, and reasonable attitudes toward the patient.

References

Davis, J. 1973. "Overdose of Psychotropic Drugs." *Psychiatric Annals* 3(4):6–11.
Donlon, P. T. and J. P. Tupin. 1977. "Successful Suicides with Thioridazine and Mesoridazine." *Archives of General Psychiatry* 34:955–77.
Dorpat, T. L. 1974. "Drug Automatism, Barbiturate Poisoning and Suicide Behavior." *Archives of General Psychiatry* 31:216–20.
FDA Drug Bulletin. 1978. 8(1):5–6.
Frederick, C., H. L. P. Resnik, and B. J. Wittlin. 1973. "Self-Destructive Aspects of Hard-Core Addiction." *Archives of General Psychiatry* 28:579–85.
Frosch, W. A., E. Robbins, and M. Stern. 1967. "Motivation for Self Administration of LSD." *Psychiatric Quarterly* 41:56–61.
Murphy, G. 1972. "Clinical Identification of Suicidal Risk." *Archives of General Psychiatry* 27:356–59.
O'Donnell, J. A. 1964. "A Follow-Up of Narcotic Addicts Mortality Relapse and Abstinence." *American Journal of Addiction* 34:948–54.
Pierce, J. I. 1967. "Suicide and Mortality Amongst Heroin Addicts in Britain." *British Journal of Addiction* 62:391–98.
Rada, R. T., R. Kellner, and J. G. Buchanan. 1975. "Chlordiazepoxide and Alcohol: A Fatal Overdose." *Journal of Forensic Sciences* 20(3):544–47.
Warren, R. D., D. S. Meuers, B. A. Paper, and J. F. Maher. 1974. "Fatal Overdose of Propoxyphene Napsylate and Aspirin: A Case Report with Pathologic and Toxiologic Study." *Journal American Medical Association* 230(2):259–60.

II.
CONTROLLING THE DYING PATIENT'S PAIN

9.
PAIN CONTROL IN THE TREATMENT OF CANCER

Ivan K. Goldberg

The pain of malignant disease varies in intensity but seldom reaches the severity of some of the other excruciating pains encountered in medical practice. It is the chronic, prolonged duration of intractable discomfort over a period of weeks or months that in time erodes the endurance of even the most resolute and creates one of the most difficult problems in pain management. The relentless downhill course with loss of weight and strength in association with continuous discomfort often results in profound emotional deterioration and increases the difficulties of patient care.

Overt pain behavior is a function of many factors: perceptual, cognitive, personality, family, and ethnic, together with the severity of the pain stimulus. It has been repeatedly shown that both anxiety and depression tend to magnify the response to a painful stimulus. Beecher pointed out that a major factor in pain is the "reaction component"—that is, the individual's perception of and reaction to the sensation of pain, including its meaning for the person, anxiety over its consequences, and so on (1959). The reaction component, he believes, is inseparable from any of the other factors contributing to the total picture of pain as experienced or pain responses. Pain-relieving drugs act on the reaction to the painful stimulus rather than on the perception of the stimulus itself. Neuroleptic (antipsychotic) drugs have been in general use for almost twenty years as a means of allowing psychotic individuals to react less strongly to their disordered thinking and perceptions. The results of studies designed to determine the usefulness of chlorpromazine for the relief of clinical pain have been inconsistent. Whereas Moore and Dundee (1961) found the analgesic potency of a mixture of antipsychotic drugs and morphine to be greater than that of morphine alone in the treatment of acute postoperative pain, Hanks et al. (1983) were unable to demonstrate that equal amounts of chlorpromazine had any potentiating action whatever on the analgesic effects of morphine when used to control the pain of hospitalized cancer patients.

Neurolepanalgesia (NLA) generally implies pain control through the simultaneous administration of a neuroleptic drug and a narcotic analgesic. The butyrophenone derivative droperidol in conjunction with the extremely rapidly acting narcotic fentanyl has most frequently been used for NLA. Whereas droperidol has a calming antianxiety action that may last as long as ten hours following the intramuscular administration of 5 mg, the analgesic properties of fentanyl usually abate after 20 or 30 minutes. However, if droperidol were to be combined with a longer acting narcotic to bring about a relaxed pain-free state in which patients are capable of responding to those around them while protected from the threat, as well as the fact, of pain, such a combination may have clinical usefulness in the management of patients with severe persistent painful conditions.

As mentioned, depression frequently intensifies the experience of pain, and a pain–depression–pain cycle may occur more frequently than is recognized. There are numerous European reports of the effectiveness of intermuscular imipramine for the relief of the severe, persistent pain frequently resulting from malignancies. Of interest is the observation in a number of these studies that imipramine is effective for pain control only after a lag period of five to ten days. (This reminds one of the seven- to fourteen-day lag period frequently seen when the drug is used as an antidepressant.) It has also been reported that the analgesic effects of imipramine are most pronounced in patients with clinical manifestations of depression. A carefully controlled double-blind clinical trial of imipramine in cancer patients with severe pain could easily clarify whether this well-tolerated drug is useful in the management of the pain of cancer.

Monoamine oxidase (MAO) inhibitors are frequently referred to as having potentiating effects on narcotics and hypnotics. A placebo-controlled double-blind study, carefully designed, may again be useful in clarifying the possible usefulness of MAO inhibitors in cancer patients. It has recently been demonstrated that 10 mg of dextroamphetamine can double the analgesic potency of morphine (Forrest et al. 1977).

A pain control team, consisting of a general surgeon, a neurosurgeon, an anesthetist, and a psychiatrist, meeting for pain rounds would be a useful way of organizing pain control services and research. The pain control team may design and carry out clinical research into such diverse innovative pain control techniques as hypnosis, LSD, nitrous oxide, analgesia, acupuncture, and other treatments of generally undetermined value.

A number of studies indicate that much more than the usual dimensions of age and sex must be considered in attempting to construct equivalent groups for clinical analgesia testing. Zborowski (1969) reports statistically significant differences between patients of old American, Irish, Italian, and Jewish backgrounds on the following dimensions: the intensity of pain, the quality of pain, the duration of pain, the description of sensation, expressive versus unexpressive behavior, tolerance of pain, attitudinal response to being in pain, attitude toward the doctor as related to pain, and attitude toward hospital care in general.

Another factor of apparent importance is Witkin's description of field dependence versus field independence (1954). A field-independent individual is one who can respond to internal clues while ignoring external distractions. Field-independent individuals have been described as more aggressive people employing more active coping behavior in dealing with the environment. They also have been found to show more psychological differentiation in their analytical responses to different stimuli. Field-dependent persons tend to be more passive and make more generalized responses to stimuli. In a study of experimental (not clinical) pain, high reactivity was associated with field independence and low pain reactivity with field dependence.

Petrie (1967) has noted a tendency in some individuals to reduce the subjective intensity of sensation after they have been stimulated by a more intense perception and the tendency by others to augment the subjective intensity of sensations. As might be expected, those people who tend subjectively to reduce the intensity of stimulation were found to tolerate pain better than others. (Of note, these same individuals were unable to tolerate sensory deprivation.) Petrie also discovered that alcohol and aspirin reduced pain only in individuals who tended to augment the intensity of stimulation. There are very few studies of the clinical behavior of augmenters or reducers suffering from clinical pain (in contrast to experimental pain).

That hypnosis can modify or abolish the experience of pain is generally accepted. Operations without pain have been repeatedly performed under hypnosis. Pilowsky and Bond (1969) have reported that even while pain is severe, the recognition of the patient's need can vary surprisingly. Using observations of patients with advanced malignant disease, they measured the patient's self-assessment of pain, the frequency of requests for medication, and the frequency with which analgesics were actually administered. It was found that analgesics were given according to patterns that were often inconsistent with the patient's own assessment of pain and with the patient's request for relief. The inconsistency was particularly marked when women were compared to men. The former received more powerful analgesics for lower pain scores, and the latter, at times, had requests for relief refused.

The schedule of administration of narcotics in the cancer patient would appear to be worth investigating further. By giving a narcotic on a regular schedule rather than waiting for a signal from the patient that the pain is becoming unbearable, it is frequently possible to reduce the anxiety of the patient and the despair and guilt of the family.

Regular doses of narcotics prevent both the threat as well as the reality of pain and relieve both anxiety and physical distress. Distress and suffering are self-reinforcing while relief leads to further relief. The use of long-acting narcotic analgesics such as methadone (Nyswander and Dole 1984) and the administration of morphine by continuous extradural infusion utilizing a microinfusion pump (Crawford et al. 1983) are ways of insuring adequate analgesia at all times.

Clinical research should lead to techniques to provide advanced cancer patients with psychic calm and freedom from pain with minimal depression of vital functions.

REFERENCES

Beecher, H. K. 1959. *Measurement of Subjective Responses: Quantitative Effects of Drugs*. New York: Oxford University Press.

Crawford, M. E. et al. 1983. "Pain Treatment on Outpatient Basis Utilizing Extradural Opiates: A Danish Multicentre Study Comprising 105 Patients." *Pain* 16:41–47.

Forrest, W. H. et al. 1977. "Dextroamphetamine with Morphine for the Treatment of Postoperative Pain." *New England Journal of Medicine* 296:712–715.

Hanks, G. W. et al. 1983. "The Myth of Haloperidol Potentiation." *Lancet* 2:523–524.

Moore, J. and J. W. Dundee. 1961. "Alterations in Response to Somatic Pain Associated with Anesthesia VII: The Effects of Nine Phenothiazine Derivatives." *British Journal of Anesthesiology* 33:422–431.

Nyswander, M. E. and V. P. Dole. 1984. "The Treatment of Chronic Pain." *New England Journal of Medicine* 296:712–715.

Petrie, A. 1967. *Individuality in Pain and Suffering*. Chicago: University of Chicago Press.

Pilowsky, I. and M. R. Bond. 1969. "Pain and Its Management in Malignant Disease: Education of Staff-Patient Transactions" *Psychological Medicine* 31:400–414.

Witkin, H. A. et al. 1954. *Personality Through Perception*. New York: Harper.

Zborowski, M. 1969. *People in Pain*. San Francisco: Jossey Bass.

10
THE USE OF DIAMORPHINE IN THE MANAGEMENT OF TERMINAL CANCER (HISTORICAL AND CHRONOLOGICAL EVOLUTION, 1971)

ROBERT G. TWYCROSS

Editors' Note: Owing to intense interest and even confusion relating to the role of diamorphine in the management of advanced cancer pain, the importance of chronologically reviewing this therapeutic modality as utilized in Great Britain is of great relevance within the context of this book. This manuscript, the *first* in this series, was presented in 1971 at The Foundation of Thanatology-sponsored Symposium, "Psychopharmacologic Agents in the Care of the Terminally Ill and the Bereaved," and was published in *Psychopharmacologic Agents for the Terminally Ill and the Bereaved,* I. K. Goldberg, S. Malitz, and A. H. Kutscher, eds., Columbia University Press, 1973. It is *not* intended to represent the state of the art in 1985.

Introduction

Diamorphine is more than just another drug; it is a phenomenon. It appears to evoke a reaction in all those who come into contact with it, whether in a truly physical way or simply via the spoken or written word.

Reactions to diamorphine, by and large, are of two types. It is described by many as one of the biggest unnatural disasters ever to hit mankind. Others, however, regard it as a powerful weapon of legitimate use, unrivaled especially in the field of terminal cancer care.

Without subscribing blindly to either view, it would be of interest to an American readership to describe the way in which diamorphine is being used in two terminal care hospitals in London. It has been used for ten years at St. Joseph's Hospice, which has 55 beds set aside for terminal cancer care, and at St. Christopher's Hospice, with approximately the same number of beds, since they opened in July 1967.

Its introduction and continuing use is largely due to the founder and Medical Director of St. Christopher's Hospice, Dr. Cicely Saunders. She noticed that, in a group of patients who vomited with a variety of other narcotics, little or no vomiting occurred after they were changed to diamorphine. Encouraged by the fact that others had also observed this (Sprott 1949; Laycock 1959), she introduced it as the treatment of choice for intractable pain in malignant disease.

However, to describe the use of diamorphine without relating such use to the total pattern of patient care at the two hospitals would almost certainly give the wrong impression. Although diamorphine may be an excellent, even unrivaled, potent analgesic, it never has been nor ever will be the answer to all the problems of terminal care.

Chronic Versus Acute Pain

It is accepted that only 40–50 percent of all cancer patients experience pain of any significance (Turnbull 1954; Aitken-Swan 1959), but because intractable pain is a common reason for hospitalization, about 70 percent of our patients on admission have pain problems and a further 5 percent develop troublesome pain during their time with us.

If one is to be successful in relieving such pain, it is of fundamental importance to appreciate that acute and chronic pain are as different from one another as acute and chronic renal failure are. It is all too easy for a physician, who in all probability has no personal experience of chronic pain, to forget this. Unfortunately for our patients, our understanding of pain is usually taken from our experience of acute pain—the toothache, the headache, the cut, or bruise. This type of pain is conducted very rapidly in the nervous system, causes defensive reflexes, and usually passes quite quickly. We are taught from childhood to regard it as a good and useful warning. Chronic pain, whether malignant or not, does not and cannot fit into such a description. It is impossible to predict when it will end. It may well go on getting worse. It appears to be utterly meaningless and causes genuine suffering. It rapidly expands to occupy the entire life field, and when that happens, life is no longer worth living. LeShan illustrates the point well:

> As the Nazis well understand and demonstrated, meaningless and purposeless torture is much harder for the person to accept and resist than is torture which the subject can place in a coherent frame of reference. A perceived senselessness in the universe weakens our belief that our efforts have validity and point. They appear to be essentially futile. This makes it much harder to continue these efforts, including those of coping with pain and stress (LeShan 1964).

Chronic pain must be thought of as consisting of three separate components: (1) Mental, (2) Social, and (3) Physical.

Undoubtedly much mental suffering is caused by the "depersonalization" that occurs in most, if not all, big hospitals. It happens so easily in a busy acute medical or surgical ward. Because there is so much to do and so little time to do it in, patients have to be regimented to enable the workload to be completed. It is very easy for the patient dying in the corner bed, possibly largely ignored, with no visits to the radiology or physiotherapy departments to provide an escape, to feel that he or she does not matter at all. Although it is the *patient's* illness, the patient is not consulted about anything, and cooperation is not sought. Resentment at everything and with everybody begins to build up, and symptoms tend to multiply and worsen—all because the patient is not being treated as a person.

At St. Christopher's and St. Joseph's we try to reverse the process. It begins at the moment a patient arrives at the door of the Hospice, where he is welcomed by a warmed bed, rather than a cold impersonal trolley, and by the Matron or deputy, who makes a point of greeting the patient by name and shaking hands: "Hello, Mr. Smith, we are very pleased to see you; we hope you will be happy with us." This might not seem at all important, but it is of great importance. It is the first step by which we hope to demonstrate that the patient matters to us and is going to be respected as a person and not just treated as a thing. The impact of the welcome can be quite extraordinary. On one occasion, a woman's symptoms of pain and general distress had virtually vanished by the time she reached the ward. On another occasion, the wife of a patient said to the Matron, as her husband was being transported to the ward, "It is marvelous to know that my husband is going to be treated as a person again." In short, a simple act of courtesy can greatly reduce anxiety and go a long way to restore a person's self-respect.

A good example of the mental aspect of pain linked with the social aspect appeared in an article in the *British Medical Journal* (1971). The article described the vocational training course for general practitioners at a center in Britain. In it was a description of the seminars that formed an integral part of the course. Patients encountered by the doctors in their routine hospital work were discussed with the help of a consultant psychiatrist, the aim being to allow the trainees to uncover psychological factors that exist even in the most apparently straightforward physical illness, and in the doctor as well. For example, one of the trainees brought to the discussion a problem of a patient with advanced bony metastases from breast cancer whose pain remained unrelieved by narcotics, whatever their type or dose. During the seminar it was suggested that the woman might be angry that neither her doctors nor relatives would admit to her she was dying or discuss all the problems created by the situation and that this was expressed in her complaints of pain. In fact, this proved to be the right explanation, and a full and frank discussion with the patient caused a dramatic improvement in her mental state and stopped her complaints of pain.

Analgesics in Cancer

Although the majority of patients with pain problems at St. Christopher's and St. Joseph's receive diamorphine, there is a minority who are maintained on a variety of other analgesics ranging from aspirin and paracetamol to dextropropoxyphene and the synthetic narcotics such as pentazocine and phenazocine. Of the majority who receive diamorphine, only 15 percent have it by injection throughout their time with us. The remainder take it as an oral mixture consisting of diamorphine 2.5 mg or more, cocaine 10 mg, ethyl alcohol (95%) 2.5 ml, syrup (66% sucrose in water) 5 ml, made up to 20 ml by the addition of chloroform water. These patients are maintained on a suitable dose given regularly every four hours to prevent the recurrence of pain. The right dose is the one that keeps the patient free of pain. With the aid of a night sedative most patients do not require a 2:00 A.M. dose, though if it is found necessary, the patient is wakened to take it rather than allowed to awaken later complaining of a recurrence of the pain. Most patients have to be transferred to parenterally administered diamorphine for the last 12–24 hours on account of increasing difficulty with swallowing or coma.

A tradition has developed whereby almost all our patients receive a phenothiazine syrup with the diamorphine mixture, usually either prochlorperazine or chlorpromazine. Originally given to relieve coexistent nausea or vomiting, it is now also given to mask the bitter taste of diamorphine. It is possible, however, that the well-documented analgesic potentiation seen with many phenothiazine derivatives accounts, at least in part, for the relatively small doses that are the norm in our hands. The contribution of the cocaine in the mixture is very much an unknown quantity.

Many patients respond dramatically to the various measures introduced on admission—measures aimed at understanding and controlling the mental, social, and physical components of chronic pain. Sometimes it may take a fortnight or more to achieve the desired result. Unfortunately, just more than 1 percent of the patients admitted with severe pain fail to obtain adequate relief, and a further 20 percent, although much relieved, do experience pain from time to time, especially when moved.

Problems Arising from Use of Diamorphine

The reasons why diamorphine rather than morphine is used at the two hospitals can be summarized as follows:

1. Diamorphine causes less nausea and vomiting than morphine.
2. The administration of diamorphine to patients with anorexia often results in a return of appetite. This is not the case with morphine.
3. Diamorphine enhances the mood of a patient, whereas morphine not infrequently causes dysphoria. This does not mean the patient becomes frankly euphoric; the improvement of mood can be seen as a return toward normal.
4. Patients on diamorphine tend to be more alert, active, and cooperative compared with patients on morphine.
5. Diamorphine is a more reliable antitussive agent.
6. Diamorphine is more effective at relieving the anxiety of patients suffering from "malignant dyspnea."

It must, however, be stated quite clearly that this is a list of supposed benefits. None has definitely been shown to be so by double-blind trial techniques in the type of patient we are concerned with. Even so, it would be unwise to disregard without question the considerable weight of clinical impression that has accumulated over a period of many years through its use mainly in the United Kingdom. Many physicians, when asked, will confirm their belief in the superiority of diamorphine.

So much for the supposed benefits of diamorphine. What of its disadvantages? These appear to be twofold:

1. High addictive potential
2. Rapid escalation of the effective dose, i.e., tolerance

When diamorphine is given prophylactically to prevent the return of otherwise intractable pain, it is very unusual to encounter true psychological addiction. Patients do not develop a craving for the drug when they no longer have to crave relief for their pain. The dangerous situation occurs when diamorphine is given on a pro re nata basis, i.e., the pain has to return before the next dose is deemed to be necessary by the nursing staff. Examples of inadequate prescribing that result in the reappearance of pain after two and one-half to three hours are not infrequently encountered both among patients referred to us and in the medical journals (Scofield 1971; *Lancet* 1971). Consequently, the patient has to endure an hour or more of agonizing pain before the next, equally inadequate, dose is given. One can understand the development of craving in such circumstances.

The other supposed danger of diamorphine—the escalation of the effective dose—is also something of a bogey. At least, it is not common in our experience. The following figures and table illustrate this point.

Table 10.1 shows the maximum doses required in a group of patients at St. Christopher's. Of the 500 patients, 438 received diamorphine, and approximately 35 percent (153/438) of these were maintained on 5 mg or less per dose until death. A further 30 percent (133/438) required no more than 10 mg. At the other end of the scale, the percentage requiring 30 mg or more per dose was about 15 percent (65/438). A breakdown of the 15 percent would show that only 4 percent (18/438) required more than 30 mg. Of these 18 patients only 4 received more than 60 mg per dose, the maximum dose being 90 mg.

Table 10.2 shows the dose scatter of a further 411 patients. Not that a higher number of patients were maintained on the lowest dose (5 mg or less). Counterbalancing this, a similar increase is seen in the high-dose column. However, the percentage of patients in the end two columns (i.e., all those receiving more

Table 10.1. Number of Patients out of Second 500 Related to the Maximum Dose of Diamorphine

Dosage	2.5	5	10	20	Over 30
Patients:	49	104	133	87	65

Table 10.2. Number of Patients out of Third 500 Related to the Maximum Dose of Diamorphine

Dosage (mg):	2.5	5	10	20	Over 30
Patients:	70	95	92	73	81

than 10 mg per dose) is approximately the same as that seen in figure 10.1, 37.5 percent as against 35 percent.

Patients are not usually given more than 40 mg of diamorphine by mouth at any one time, for experience suggests that, above this level, increase in dose is not always followed by an appropriate increase in analgesia.

In conclusion, there are many other techniques that should, in certain situations, be employed, either with or without the concurrent use of narcotics, ranging from diversional activity to neurosurgery (see table 10.3). Their use can be summarized in the words of Professor Ritchie Russell:

Table 10.3. Additional Analgesic Measures

Psychological	Diversional activity
	Antidepressants
Pharmacological	Tranquilizers
	Steroids
	Cytotoxic drugs
Physical	Refrigerant spray
	Local heat
	Fixation
	Jobst decompression
	Sensory blockade
Injections	Local anaesthetic
	Peripheral nerve block
	Autonomic nerve block
	Intrathecal block
Neurosurgery	Leucotomy
	Hypophysectomy
	Peripheral nerve section
	Cordotomy
Palliative surgery	
Irradiation	
Biochemical	
Thermotherapy	
Hypnosis	

I would suggest that the successful therapist for intractable pain treats the problem like a game in which he endeavours to outmanoeuvre the tricks performed by the central nervous system of his patient. He has many different moves he can play. Some depend on simple procedures which checkmate the mechanisms, but others are assisted by the deception of the poker player and the confidence of the quack (Russell 1959).

References

Aitken-Swan, J. 1959. "Nursing the Late Cancer Patient at Home. The Family's Impressions." *Practitioner* 183:64.
Editorial. 1971. "Understanding Pain." *Lancet* 1:1284.
From a Special Correspondent. 1971. "Vocational Training for General Practice. 1. A District Hospital's Scheme: Ipswich."*British Medical Journal* 2:704.
Laycock, J. D. 1959. "Pain Relieving Drugs." *St. Thomas's Hospital Gazette* 5–7:10.
LeShan, L. 1964. "The World of the Patient in Severe Pain of Long Duration." *Journal of Chronic Diseases* 17:119.
Russell, W. R. 1959. "Discussion on the Treatment of Interactable Pain." *Proceedings of the Royal Society of Medicine* 52:983.
Scofield, P. B. 1971. "Analgesics in Terminal Disease." *British Medical Journal* 2:773.
Sprott, N. A. 1949. "Dying of Cancer." *Medical Press and Circular* 221:197.
Turnbull, F. 1954. "Intractable Pain." *Proceedings of the Royal Society of Medicine* 47:155.

11.
THE USE AND ABUSE OF NARCOTIC ANALGESICS IN TERMINAL CANCER (HISTORICAL AND CHRONOLOGICAL EVOLUTION, 1974)

ROBERT G. TWYCROSS

Editors' Note: **Owing to intense interest and even confusion relating to the role of diamorphine in the management of advanced cancer pain, the importance of chronologically reviewing this therapeutic modality as utilized in Great Britain is of great relevance within the context of this book. This manuscript, the** *second* **in this series, is published here for the first time. It was presented in 1974 at The Foundation of Thanatology-sponsored Symposium, "Acute Grief and the Funeral." It is** *not* **intended to represent the state of the art in 1985.**

Anxiety and confusion surround the use of narcotic analgesics. Fear of addiction or the rapid escalation of the effective dose has led to underprescribing—too little being given too late or not at all. Muddled thinking, due to a failure to distinguish between different situations, has led to unwarranted generalizations about the advantages and disadvantages of the various preparations. In addition, there is a dearth of reliable data concerning the effects of narcotic analgesics when given by mouth on a long-term basis. This has resulted in considerable misuse of these drugs by the medical profession. The purpose of this article is to emphasize the need for clearer thinking, a greater appreciation of the nature of pain, more clinical trials, and a reconsideration of some of the popular beliefs concerning narcotic analgesics.

Areas of Confusion

In considering narcotic analgesics, it is important to distinguish between postoperative and terminal cancer pain, between the effects of a single dose and those of multiple repeated doses, between parenteral and oral usage, between the addict and the nonaddict, and, also, between animal experiments and studies in man. It cannot be assumed that conclusions derived from observations in one situation are necessarily valid for the others. For example, it is generally considered that 30 mg of pentazocine is equianalgesic with 10 mg of morphine. This figure is derived from a comparison of *peak* analgesic effect in postoperative patients. However, if total analgesic effects are compared, the potency ratio increases to approximately 1:4 (Paddock et al. 1969), while, in cancer patients, the equivalent ratio is 1:6 (Beaver et al. 1966). Further, by mouth, pentazocine hardly counts as a potent analgesic: two single-dose trials compared orally administered pentazocine 50 mg with, in the first, codeine 65 mg, aspirin 650 mg, and paracetamol 650 mg and, in the second, aspirin 1000 mg combined with codeine 16 mg and paracetamol 650 mg combined with propoxyphene 65 mg (Moertal et al. 1972; Robbie and Samarasinghe 1973). In the former, no significant difference was noted among the four drugs, and in the latter the aspirin-codeine combination was shown to be superior to both paracetamol-propoxyphene and pentazocine. One is led to conclude that "pentazocine is of somewhat limited use in the control of chronic pain" (WHO 1972)—a far cry from the enthusiastic support originally given to this preparation.

Chronic Pain

Pain is a psychobiologic phenomenon; that is, apart from its anatomic and physiologic components, it has a psychologic aspect. Failure to appreciate this can limit the degree of pain relief obtainable with narcotic analgesics (Twycross 1972). Chronic pain differs from acute pain in a number of ways: it is a situation rather than an event. Unlike acute pain it is impossible to predict when it will end; it tends to get worse rather than better; it appears to be entirely meaningless and, frequently, expands rapidly to occupy the entire life-field. Thus there is a greater likelihood of a negative (pain-potentiating) psychologic component in chronic pain than in acute pain. The variation in the therapeutic equivalence of pentazocine serves to emphasize the clinical difference between the two kinds of pain.

Pain due to advancing cancer is usually continuous even if variable in intensity. Because the pain is continuous, treatment should also be continuous—that is, prophylactic or preventive rather than *pro re nata* or "as required." Since pain is itself, perhaps, the most potent antianalgesic, allowing the pain to reemerge before administering the next dose both causes unnecessary suffering and encourages clinical tolerance.

Areas of Anxiety

Many physicians are reluctant, to prescribe narcotic analgesics regularly even in patients with incurable cancer, on account of fears of addiction, rapid escalation of dose, and impairment of patients' mental faculties. However, if one searches the literature for data relating to the incidence and severity of these symptoms in clinical practice, one finds that virtually none exist. In order to help correct this deficiency, it was decided in 1974 to review retrospectively 500 patients with advanced cancer admitted consecutively to St. Christopher's Hospice (London). In such patients, diamorphine is given as the narcotic analgesic of choice for severe pain. In addition, it is occasionally prescribed for distressing cough or dyspnea or for general discomfort when other measures have failed.

About 15 percent of the patients for whom diamorphine is prescribed receive it either predominantly or exclusively by injection; the rest receive it by mouth in an elixir containing both diamorphine and cocaine.* It is administered regularly every four hours in order to achieve and maintain pain relief. The initial dose of diamorphine is usually 2.5–10 mg; this is adjusted as necessary until effective analgesia is obtained. The dose of cocaine, however, is not altered. With the aid of a night sedative many patients do not require a dose at 1 A.M., though, if necessary, patients are wakened to have further medication rather than allow them to wake up later complaining of pain. Ultimately, most patients are transferred to parenterally administered diamorphine for the last 12 to 24 hours on account of increasing debility; the dose given is half the previous satisfactory oral one. Virtually all patients receiving diamorphine also receive a phenothiazine—for example, prochlorperazine, promazine, or chlorpromazine—primarily to control or prevent nausea and vomiting but also for sedation and analgesic potentiation. Other drugs, such as glucocorticosteroids, tranquilizers, and antidepressants, are also prescribed when indicated.

Retrospective Review

Of the 500 patients reviewed, 282 (56 percent) were women 218 (44 percent) were men. Median survival for the women was twenty days, for the men twelve. The age distribution is shown in table 11.1. Their diagnoses covered the whole range of malignant disease, with carcinoma of the breast and of the bronchus accounting for nearly 40 percent of the total. Of the 500 patients, 418 (84 percent) received diamorphine for varying lengths of the time.

In order to obtain a general impression of the quantities used, a maximum-dose histogram was constructed (fig. 11.1). From it we see that more than 60 percent of these patients were maintained on 10 mg per dose or less and only 8 percent required

Table 11.1 Age Distribution of the 500 Patients

Age in Years	Number of Patients
<30	5
30–39	14
40–49	40
50–59	118
60–69	174
70–79	117
>80	32
Total	500

more than 30 mg/dose. Unfortunately these figures take no account either of the route of administration or the duration of treatment. Since, however, the maximum oral dose used was 40 mg, all the patients represented in the more than 40 mg/dose column received such doses by injection—eleven patients requiring 50 or 60 mg and three 90 mg—and some six to ten patients represented in the other columns also received their maximum dose by injection.

The time factor was introduced, initially, by dividing the patients into short- and long-term survivors (up to two weeks and more than two weeks) and also into low- and high-dose groups (up to 10 mg and more than 10 mg). Significantly more of the short-term survivors required only low doses of diamorphine, whereas significantly more of the long-term survivors required high doses (table 11.2). It seems, therefore, that the amount of diamorphine required to control a patient's pain increases with time.

In order to examine the rate of increase in dose of diamorphine, the patients were grouped according to survival, excluding the 213 who died within a week of commencing treatment (table 11.3). The *final daily dose* was recorded for each patient: this was defined as the median daily dose given during the last four weeks of treatment in group 5, the last complete week of treatment in group 3 and 4, and the last three days of the last complete week of treatment in groups 1 and 2. The median final daily dose for each group was then determined and, in order to correct for time, divided by the group median duration of treatment. The rate of increase in dose becomes progressively less the longer the duration of treatment.

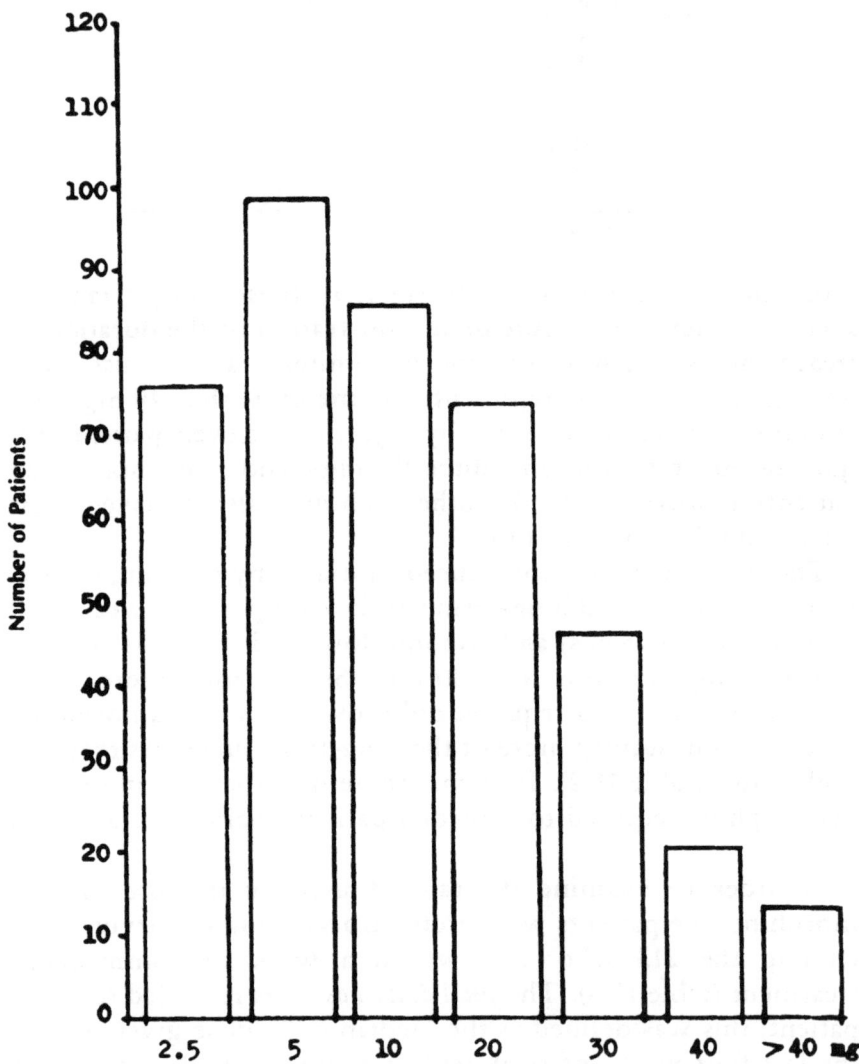

Figure 11.1. Histogram of Maximum Doses of Diamorphine

It was decided next to examine in detail those patients who survived six months after beginning treatment with diamorphine (table 11.4). All 13 patients were given a phenothiazine concurrently, 11 were prescribed prednisone (5 mg tid), and

Table 11.2 The Maximum Dose of Diamorphine Related to Duration of Treatment

	Number of Patients in Each Group		
Dose	≤2 weeks	>2 weeks	Total
Low (≤10 mg)	194	67	261
High (>10 mg)	43	114	157
Total	237	181	418

$x^2 = 88 \ (\nu = 1)$
$p < .001$

eight required an antidepressant during the major part of their treatment. In addition, six received a nonnarcotic analgesic for varying lengths of time. None of the patients required a steady, relentless increase in dose. In two cases the graph was like a plateau (figs. 11.3, 11); in three "crescendo-diminuendo" (figs. 11.9, 13, 14), and undulating in three more (figs. 11.2, 4, 8). In the remaining five patients the pattern was one of multiple plateau separated by steps, but in only one of these (fig. 11.10) were all the steps in an upward direction. The question suggested by these case histories is *does the diamorphine have to be increased because of tolerance or because of increasing pain?*

In Case 1 the dose of diamorphine undulated. Several of the upward adjustments in the dose of diamorphine were for pain associated with different metastatic lesions. This fact, coupled with the subsequent dose decreases, suggests that, in this patient at least, increases in diamorphine were made because of increased pain rather than because of tolerance.

In Case 3, where the dose chart shows three elevations, the first and third relate to clearly defined episodes. In both, a new

Table 11.3 Assessment of the Rate of Increase in Dose of Diamorphine in 205 Patients Who Received Diamorphine for One Week or More

Number of complete weeks	1	2–3	4–7	8–15	≥16
Number of patients	58	39	53	34	21
Median final daily dose (mg)	50	60	95	125	135
Median duration of treatment (weeks)	1.5	3	6	12	24
Dose-Time	33	20	16	10	6

Note: The figures in the bottom row are obtained by dividing the group median final daily dose in mg by the group median duration of treatment in weeks.

Table 11.4. Summarized Data Relating to the Thirteen Patients Who Were Alive Twenty-Four Weeks After Starting Treatment with Diamorphine

Case No.	Sex	Age	Primary Site of Carcinoma	Duration of Treatment with Diamorphine (Weeks)	Initial Clinical Condition	Subsequent Course of Events
1	F	64	Breast	99	Bedfast, nauseated, and anorexic; weight loss; severe pain in back and right leg.	Nausea and pain gradually controlled, appetite returned to normal. Fully mobile after two months. Subsequently discharged but readmitted several times on account of pain and/or depression. Inpatient for last ten weeks. Mood variable during this time. Diamorphine administered parenterally for last five weeks because of a recurrence of pain.
2	M	65	Lung*	76	Activity extremely limited by exertional dyspnea. Also troubled by pleuritic pain. Worried and anxious; poor appetite.	Initial treatment included diamorphine, prednisone, and antibiotics. He steadily improved, became pain-free, and began to occupy himself doing carpentry. Was discharged after six months but subsequently admitted to another hospital for reinvestigation, where the diamorphine was rapidly tailed off. However, owing to withdrawal symptoms this was restarted. The patient died from an acute respiratory infection five months later.
3	F	62	Breast	50	In pain, nausea, some vomiting. Subsequent worsening of pain. Able to walk with crutches.	Became fully mobile, despite pain from fresh metastatic activity. Eventually able to go home for over three months. Finally readmitted with pneumonia and died within hours.

4	F	47	Caecum	Distressed, tearful, in pain, vomiting.	Improved as symptoms controlled. Troubled by recurrence of pain. Became depressed after about five months. Responded to imipramine. Readmitted four weeks before death. Required parenteral diamorphine to control pain.
5	F	44	Breast	Frightened. Complaining of nausea and vomiting, intermittent pain. Bedfast, paraplegic.	Pain, nausea, and vomiting brought under control. Mood variable—had major family problems. Latterly drowsy most of the time. Slept for long periods. Died peacefully of pneumonia.
6	F	71	Breast	Too weak to walk. Severe pain developed one week after admission and led to prescription of diamorphine.	Gradually improved. Able to walk with frame. Diamorphine stopped for three weeks. Patient discharged twice—for four months on the second occasion. Readmitted because of bad back pain—diamorphine increased. Subsequently steady till death two months later.
7	M	62	Lung*	Severe abdominal pain, anorexia, malaise. Occasional nausea and vomiting. Recent marked deterioration with massive hepatomegaly.	Pain and vomiting slowly controlled. Became fully mobile and felt generally better. Discharged after six weeks and, apart from a period of two weeks, remained at home until two days before his death, over six months later.
8	M	70	Prostrate	Depressed by constant pain in thoracic spine, pelvis, and other bones. Complained of insomnia, anorexia, and weight loss. Able to walk a little.	Became free of pain, fully mobile, ate and slept normally. Felt exceptionally well. Discharged after seven weeks. At home for 4½ months, gradually weakening latterly. Readmitted and died after one week.

Case No.	Sex	Age	Primary Site of Carcinoma	Duration of Treatment with Diamorphine (Weeks)	Initial Clinical Condition	Subsequent Course of Events
9	M	75	Rectum	27	In severe pain, limited to bed and chair.	Cancer pain controlled, arthritic pain alleviated. Gradually mobilized. Discharged after two months to care of a friend. Readmitted after only five weeks—strain too much for friend. She died three months later.
10	F	69	Stomach	24	Able to walk. Tense and anxious, in severe epigastric and back pain. Complained of nausea, marked anorexia, weight loss.	Became completely free of pain, appetite restored. Fully mobile and able to help on the ward. Discharged three weeks after beginning diamorphine. Able to stay at home for five months. Deteriorated latterly, readmitted, and died of pneumonia three days later.
11	F	64	Ovary	24	Although weak and tired, able to walk a little. In severe epigastric and back pain. Complained of anorexia, nausea, and vomiting.	Pain controlled adequately though required diamorphine by injection after about five weeks. Vomiting controlled, though this required changes in treatment. Never became fully mobile. Variable degree of alertness and activity; cheerful when alert.
12	F	56	Breast	24	Bedfast; in severe pain in both thighs, hips, and left pelvis. Nausea, anorexia. Paranoid and depressed.	Fully mobile and pain-free. Psychiatric state required constant surveillance. Diamorphine eventually discontinued and patient discharged for five months. Terminal phase probably precipitated by cessation of prednisone: fairly rapid deterioration over several weeks with evidence of renewed secondary activity.

| 13 | F | 16 | Osteosarcoma | 15 | Severe pain left groin and calf. Discharging biopsy wound. Marked anorexia and nausea. Incontinent of urine, very frightened, withdrawn. | Required increasing doses of diamorphine as mobilized. Eventually tailed off in view of remission. A limp due to left leg shortening only residuum. Alive and well three years later. |

*Later rediagnosed as "pulmonary shadowing of unknown cause."

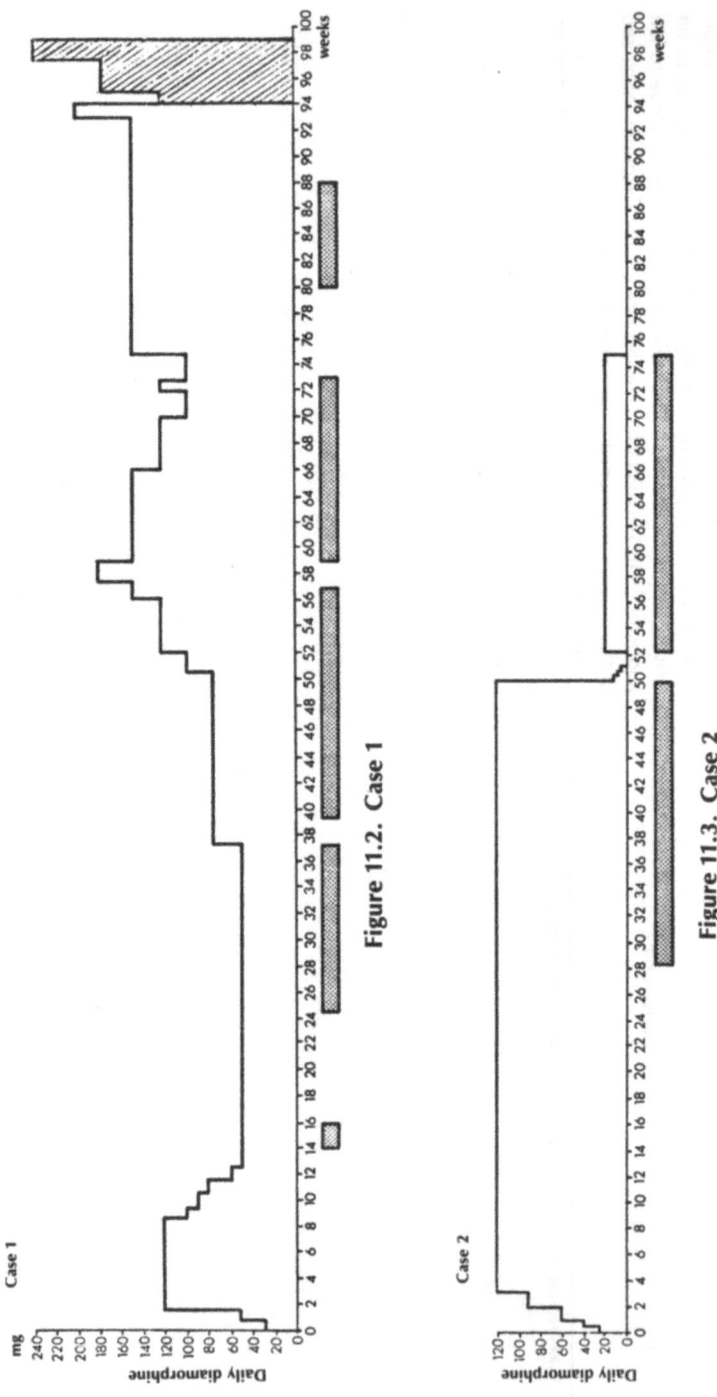

Figure 11.2. Case 1

Figure 11.3. Case 2

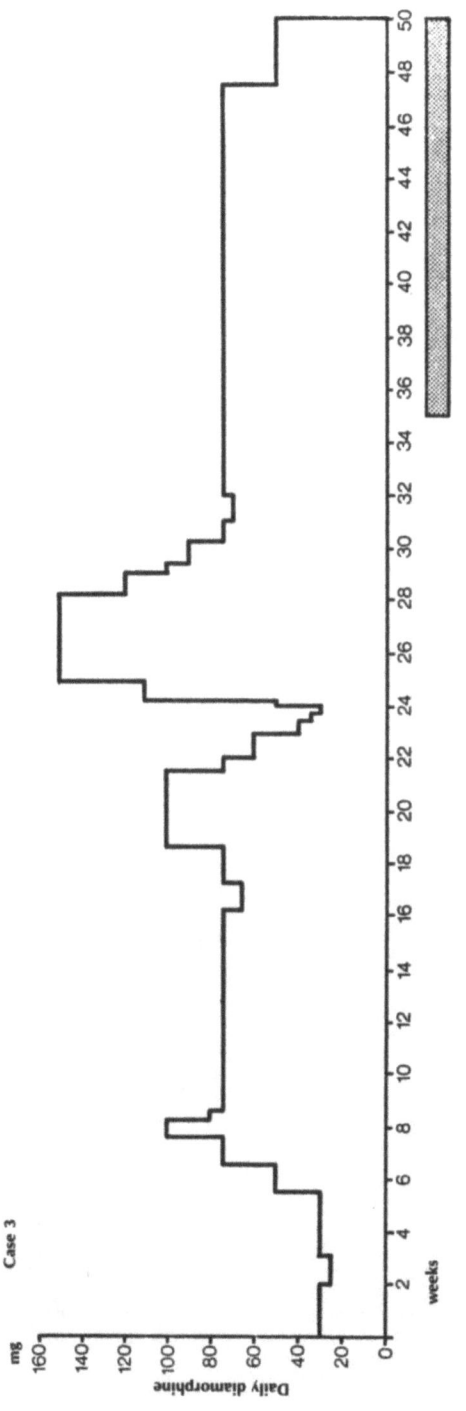

Figure 11.4. Case 3

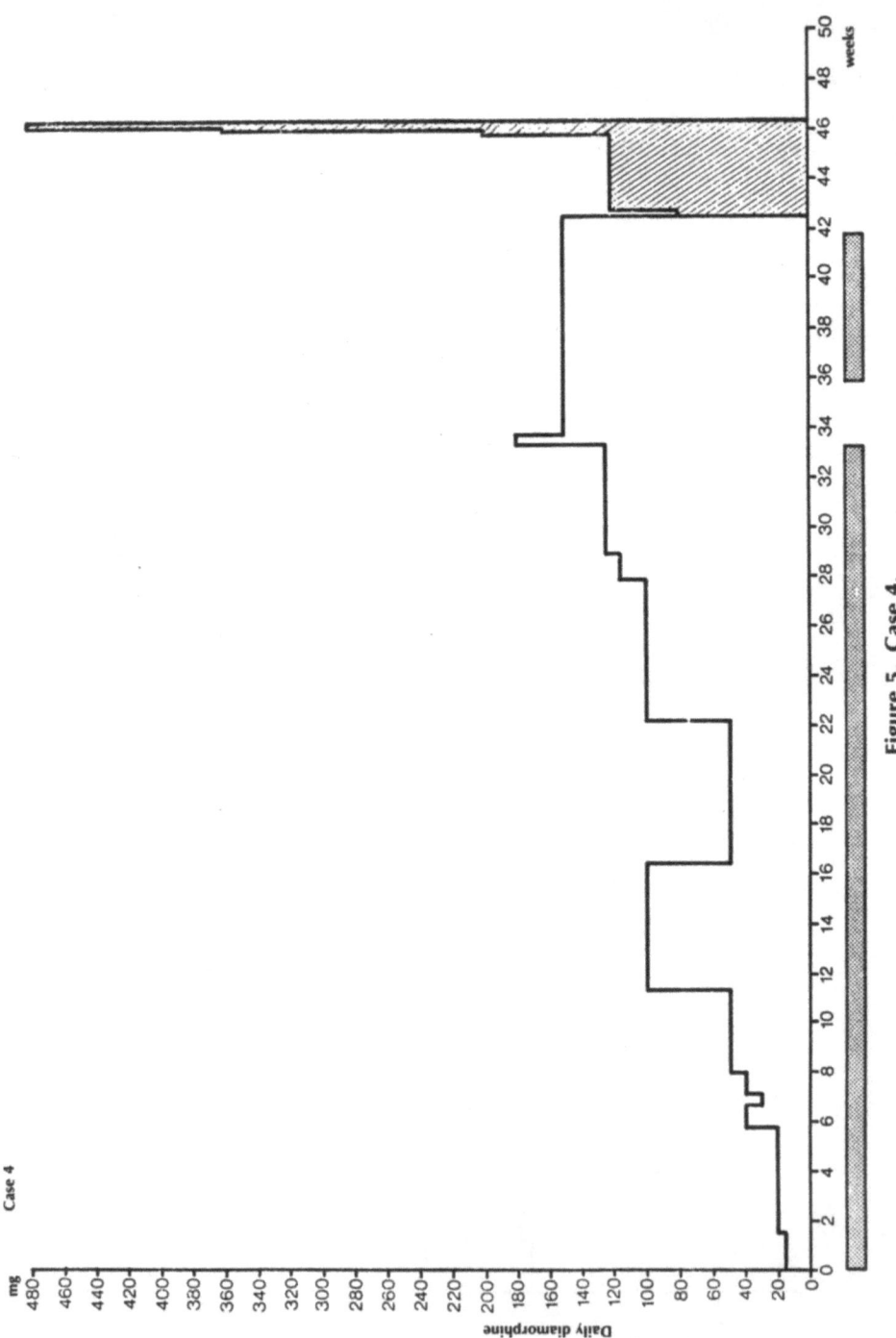

Figure 5. Case 4.

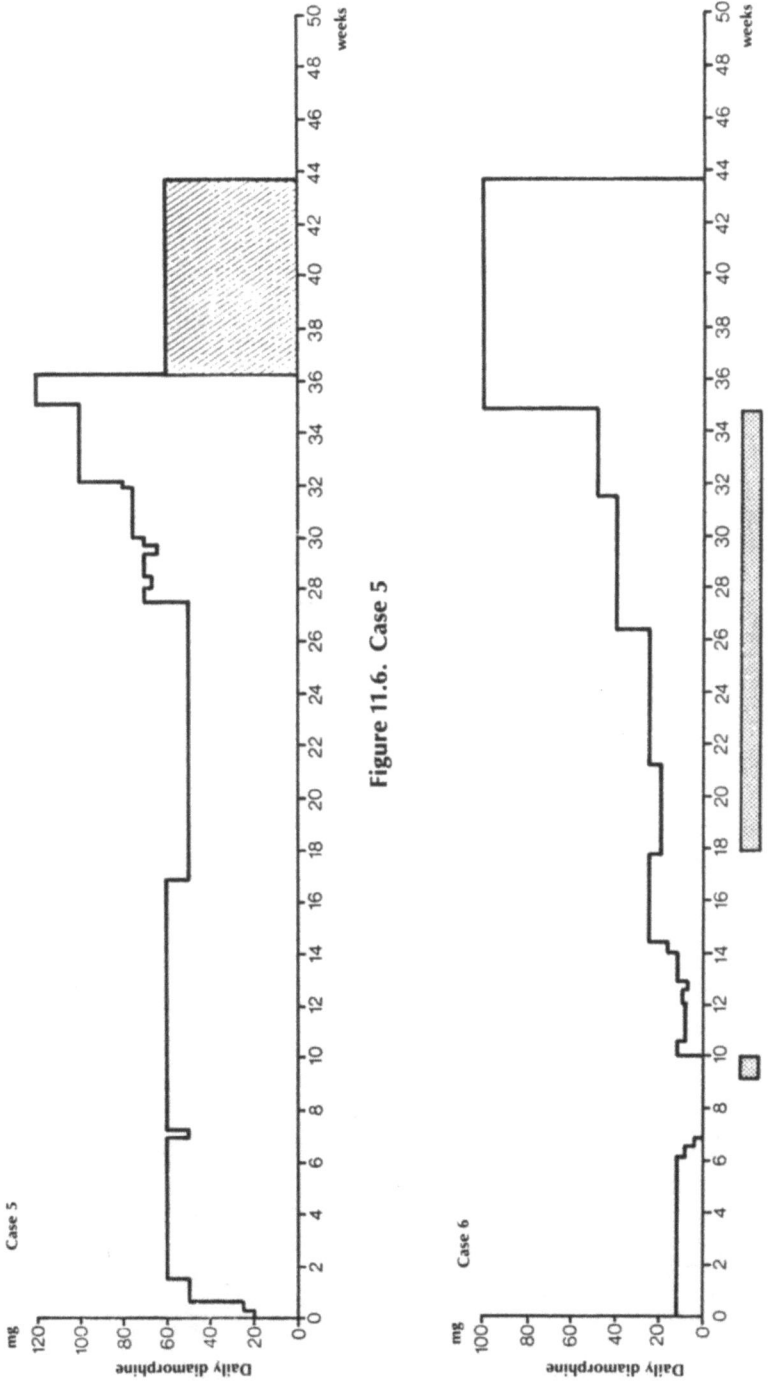

Figure 11.6. Case 5

Figure 11.7. Case 6

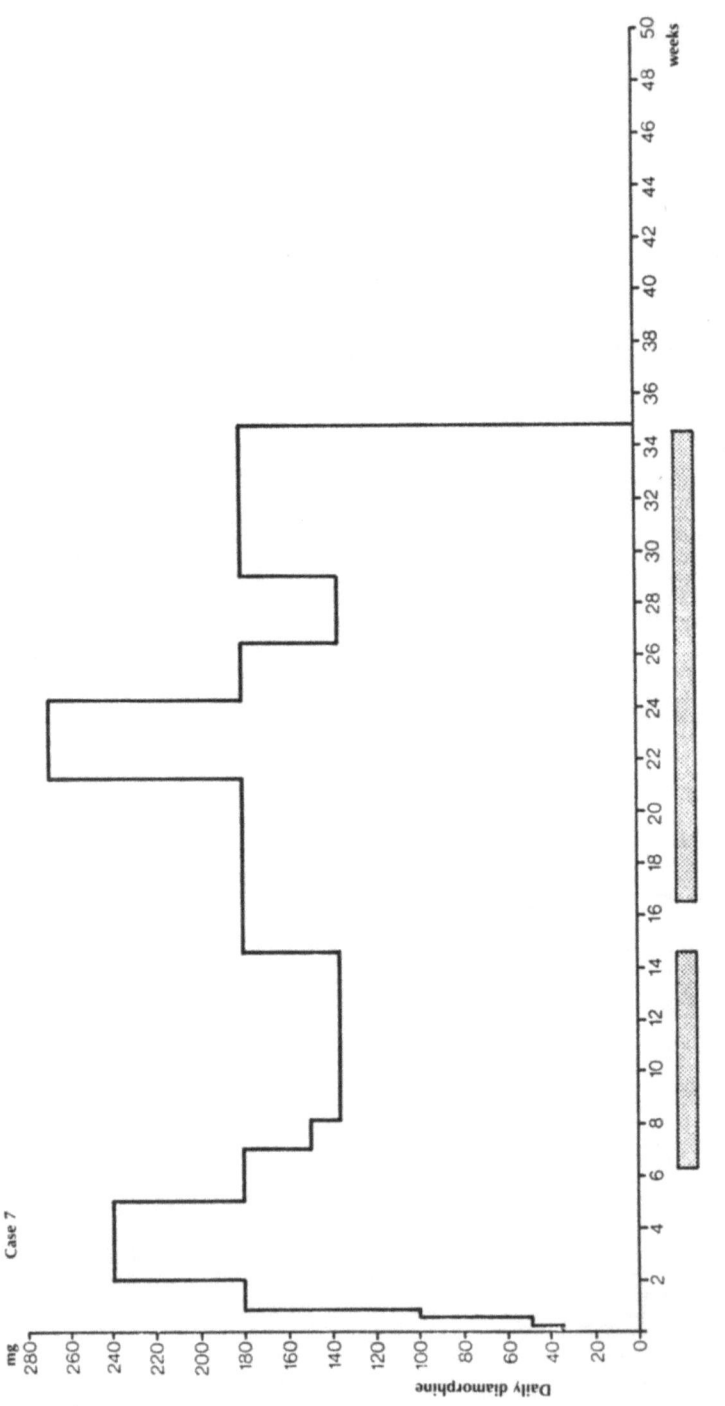

Figure 11.8. Case 7

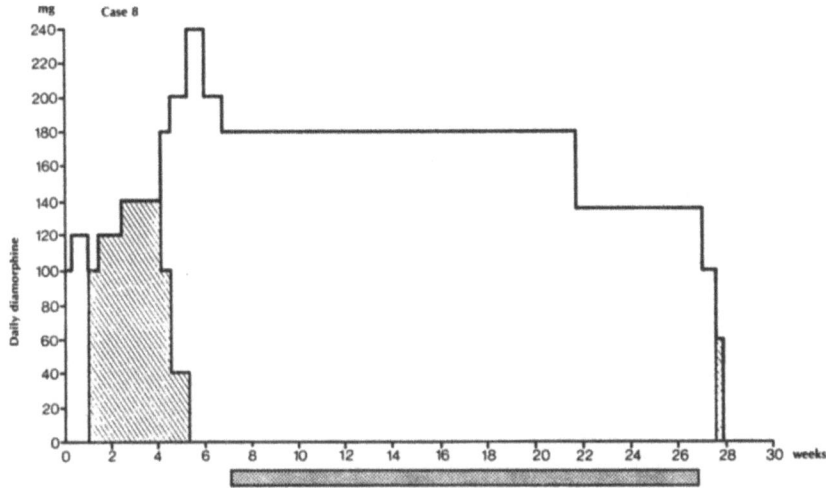

Figure 11.9. Case 8

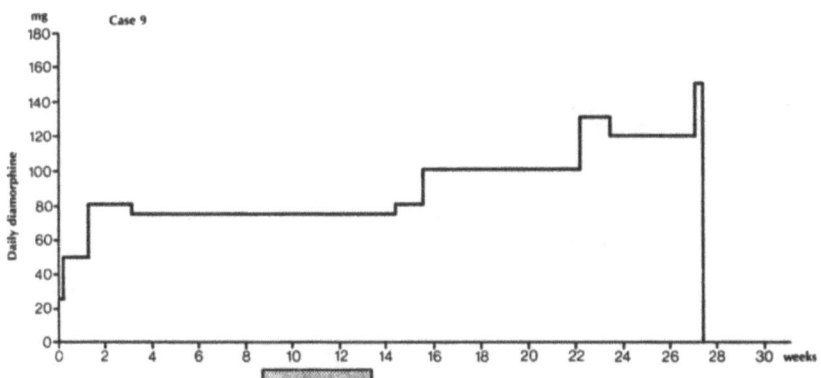

Figure 11.10. Case 9

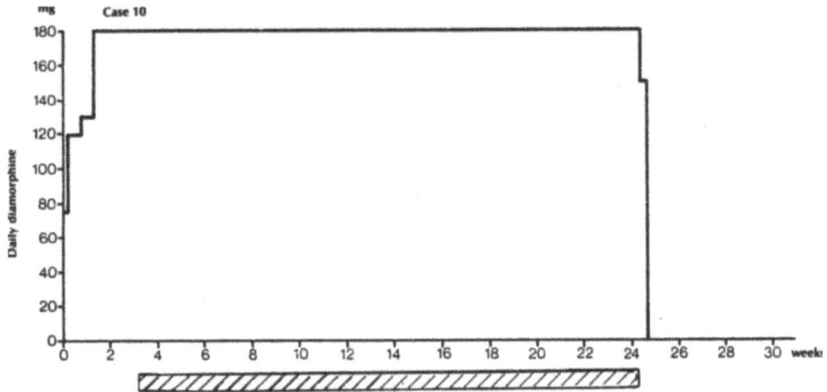

Figure 11.11. Case 10

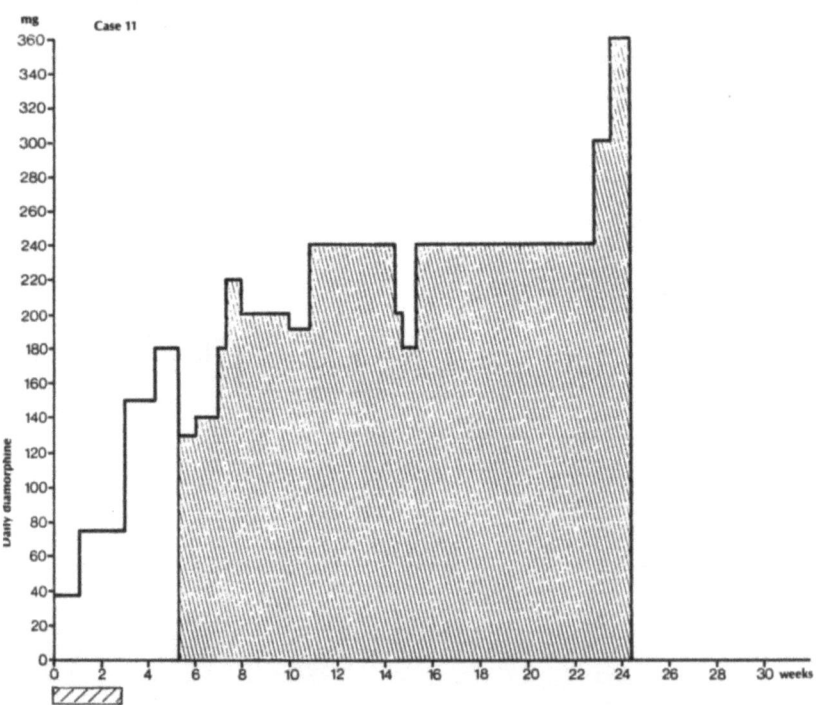

Figure 11.12. Case 11

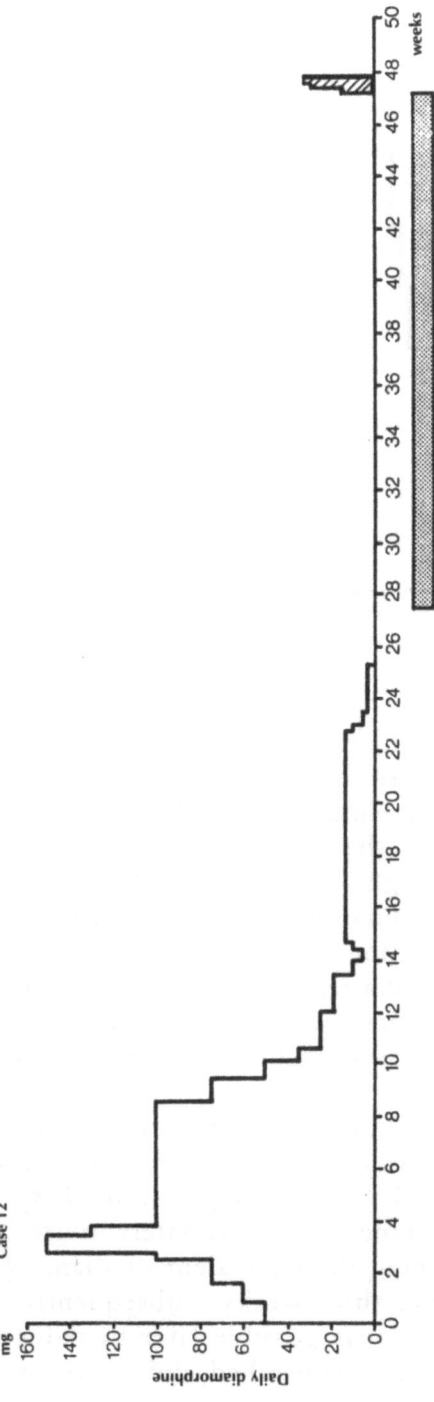

Figure 11.13. Case 12

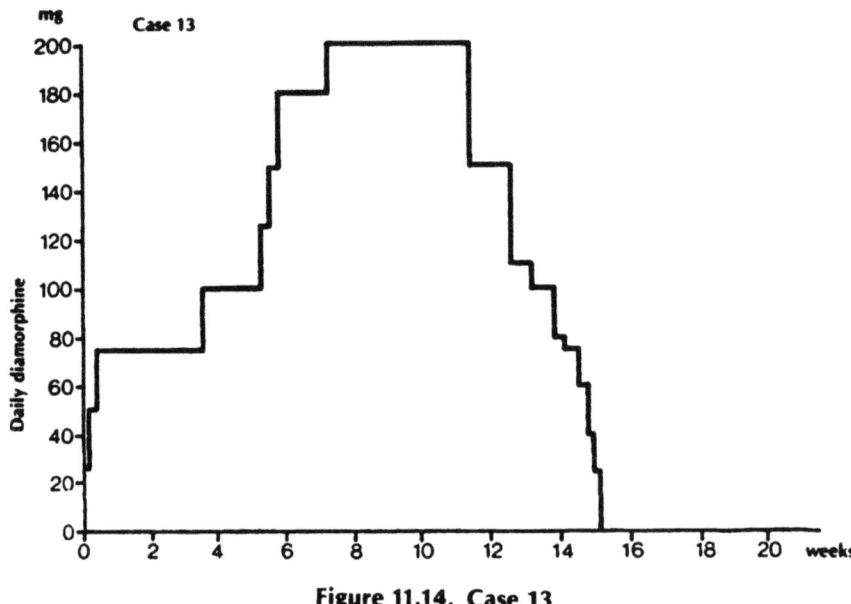

Figure 11.14. Case 13

pain caused by fresh metastatic activity precipitated the increased requirement. In the second elevation, the recurrence of a previous pain led to the increase. At first sight, then, tolerance to diamorphine might be suspected. However, the ability to make a fourfold reduction in dose some three weeks later suggests that this elevation also resulted from an acute episode relating to a bony metastasis. The final reduction, made by the patient's general practitioner, led to recurrence of intermittent discomfort, demonstrating that the patient still required analgesia at this stage.

Case 8 is notable in that the patient required diamorphine by injection during the early part of treatment because of poor control of pain with the oral preparation. If we accept that by injection diamorphine is approximately twice as potent, this patient was receiving the equivalent of diamorphine 280 mg/day by mouth after three weeks. Subsequently, he reverted to oral therapy, and it was possible later to reduce the dose still further. The pain, once controlled, did not recur apart from one or two isolated occasions. In Cases 12 and 13 it was possible to curtail treatment with diamorphine completely, the reduction in dose being linked to reduction in pain. Neither patient experienced symptoms attributable to withdrawal of diamorphine.

Case 11 emphasizes that treatment by injection is not incompatible with relatively long survival. It also reinforces the fact that, in our experience, only the minority of patients require parenteral treatment for any length of time.

In Case 10, the patient was discharged after only three weeks, having been admitted with severe epigastric pain. The diamorphine was not increased during the five months she was at home despite the diagnosis of progressive carcinoma of the stomach. Case 2 was the other instance of a prolonged plateau-like dose-time graph. This patient was prescribed diamorphine more for general distress and dyspnea than for pain. A year after beginning treatment he was admitted to another hospital for further investigation. The dose of diamorphine was immediately reduced to a tenth of its previous level without precipitating withdrawal symptoms. These appeared only when the diamorphine was completely stopped ten days later. Whether or not a less hasty termination of treatment would have prevented the appearance of the withdrawal symptoms is an open question. The outcome in Cases 12 and 13 suggests that the answer is in the affirmative.

Discussion and Conclusions

A number of conclusions may be drawn from these data.

1. *The prescription of diamorphine does not, by itself, lead to impairment of mental faculties.* It has been suggested that administration of a potent narcotic analgesic to patients with inoperable cancer is like sentencing them "to a kind of living death" (Bunyard 1971). Others speak of "detachment from reality" or imply that patients receiving morphine or diamorphine can do little more than lie "drugged" in bed. However, my own experience from treating several hundred patients with diamorphine is that this is not so. Indeed, in the present series of 500 patients, forty-six were discharged for varying lengths of time, and of

these twenty-two were on diamorphine at the time of discharge. These patients were alert and mobile, though one or two of the more elderly ones required a walking frame. Their diamorphine requirements ranged from 2.5 to 30 mg. four-hourly—that is, up to 150 mg of diamorphine a day by mouth. This suggests that "detachment from reality"—if it occurs—and drowsiness are related more to advanced physical debility than to the diamorphine.

2. *Tolerance is not a practical problem.* The data in this review, especially those relating to patients who survived for 24 weeks or more after commencing treatment with diamorphine, support the hypothesis that increases in dose are caused more by increased pain than by tolerance. It is, of course, possible to induce marked tolerance by needlessly increasing the dose (Fraser et al. 1957). However, there is certainly no foundation for the statement that because of tolerance, morphine is no longer effective after three months of continuous use (Milton 1972). In practice, when diamorphine is used as at St. Christopher's—regularly, prophylactically, and as part of a program of total patient care—tolerance, if it occurs, is not a practical problem.

3. *Psychological dependence does not occur.* Drug dependence (addiction) is defined as:

> A state, psychic and sometimes also physical, resulting from the interaction between a living organism and a drug, characterised by behavioral and other responses that always include a compulsion to take the drug on a continuous or periodic basis in order to experience its psychic effects, and sometimes to avoid the discomfort of its absence. Tolerance may or may not be present. [World Health Organization 1969].

This is a broader definition than that of 1964, which emphasized the need for both tolerance and an early development of physical dependence in addition to strong psychic dependence (World Health Organization 1964). The term *drug dependence* now more closely approximates to the popular conception of addiction—a compulsion or overpowering drive to take the drug in order to experience its psychic effects. According to this definition, none of the patients reviewed became addicted. Occasionally a patient has been admitted to the Hospice who has appeared to be addicted. Such a patient typically has a long history of poor pain control, is receiving fairly regular ("q4h prn") but inadequate injections of a narcotic analgesic, and demands an injection every two or three hours. Usually, with time and patience, it is possible to control the pain adequately, prevent clock-watching and demanding behavior, and sometimes even transfer patients onto an oral preparation. But even here, can it be said that the patient is truly addicted? Is he craving the narcotic in order to experience its psychic effects or, what is more likely, relief from pain for at least one or two hours?

4. *Physical dependence is not a problem.* It is possible but by no means certain that many of the 205 patients who received diamorphine for more than one week became physically dependent on it: dependence was clearly demonstrated after a year in Case 2. In 1959 Eddy and his associates (1959) published a review of cancer patients maintained on subcutaneous morphine, oxymorphone, and anileridine. They tested for physical dependence by injecting nalorphine hydrochloride 1 mg subcutaneously at fortnightly intervals. They were able to show that over half the patients had developed physical dependence by the end of the second week of treatment and that it was unusual for a patient not to be physically dependent by the end of the fourth week. All the patients were, however, receiving morphine by injection, whereas, according to Lee (1942), when the drug is administered by mouth, dependence develops less rapidly and possibly to a lesser degree. Even so, whether or not physical dependence develops, it does not prevent the gradual downward adjustment of dose or the complete curtailment of treatment when this becomes clinically feasible.

5. *Oral medication is adequate in the majority of cases.* Of our 500 patients, 85 percent were maintained on oral therapy until death or until the last twelve to twenty-four hours before death, when increasing debility made oral administration difficult if not impossible. The main reason for parenteral administration at an earlier stage was unrelieved nausea and vomiting. Nowadays, with a wide range of synthetic narcotic analgesics available in tablet and suppository form, doctors are well acquainted with the fact that alimentary administration is usually adequate. However, for many doctors, the prescription of morphine or diamorphine is still equated with injections. This review demonstrates that this is not so as far as diamorphine is concerned: unpublished data indicate that morphine is also effective by mouth.

6. *The optimal dose varies considerably.* In 1954 Lasagna and Beecher defined the optimal dose of a drug as that which provides the desired therapeutic effects with a minimum of undesirable side effects. A study of the dose-response curve for morphine administered intramuscularly in postoperative patients led them to conclude that the optimal dose was 10 mg per 70 kg body weight. Although one cannot disagree with their definition, it is incorrect to equate the dose above which the dose-response curve begins to flatten with "optimal dose." The optimal doses of diamorphine in the patients reviewed ranged

from as little as 2.5 mg by mouth to 90 mg by injection, the latter being equivalent to some 200 mg of intramuscular morphine.

In the light of these comments it should be possible to agree on a basis for the logical use of analgesics in terminal cancer pain.

AIM
To keep the patient both free of pain and fully alert.

METHOD

1. *Chronic pain* demands preventive therapy, which means that analgesics should be given regularly and prophylactically: "prn" is both irrational and inhumane.

2. *The right dose* is that which gives relief for a reasonable period of time: a four-hourly interval should be regarded as the norm between administrations.

3. *Nonnarcotic analgesics* should be tried in the first instance.

4. *If ineffective, transfer to a stronger preparation.*

5. *Establish a simple, analgesic "league table"* (table 11.5). "Morphine exists to be given, not merely to be withheld."

6. *Adjuvant medication* is the rule rather than the exception. A phenothiazine such as prochlorperazine or chlorpromazine acts as an antiemetic and, possibly, potentiates analgesia.

7. *Use oral medication whenever possible;* it is easier to administer and gives the patient a greater degree of freedom.

8. *There is more to analgesia than analgesics.* Some pain responds better to other forms of treatment—for example, radiotherapy, cytotoxic drugs, nerve blocks, alone or in combination with analgesics.

9. *Diversional therapy.* The perception of pain requires both attention and consciousness. Diversional therapy—people to talk to, activities to attend, and so on—is, therefore, of great value.

10. *Diamorphine/morphine must not be regarded as a panacea.* The use of these drugs does not guarantee success, particularly if the psychologic component of pain is ignored.

Table 11.5. Analgestic League Table

1. Morphine/levorphanol/methadone
2. Intermediate-strength synthetics
   (e.g., hydromorphone, dipipanone)
3. Codeine/propoxyphene ± 4
4. Aspirin/acetaminophen

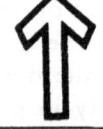 Increasing potency

Note. 1. This is not intended to be exhaustive.
2. Pethidine and pentazocine have been omitted because both are unreliable by mouth and relatively short-acting by injection.

There is a great need for further clinical trials and related research. The benefit of the cocaine in the traditional cocktail calls for evaluation, and the complex and complicating role of prednisone requires elucidation. For example, in Case 1 it is highly likely that the patient was hypercalcemic when admitted: she improved steadily once prednisone was prescribed. Hypercalcemia is known to precipatate or exacerbate pain in malignant disease and its correction to cause relief (Galasko and Burn, 1971). It is possible that alteration of the biochemical milieu in other ways can alter the pain threshold and thus a patient's narcotic requirement. Yet although many questions remain unanswered, if diamorphine can be regarded as a model, it would seem that certain beliefs concerning the use of narcotic analgesics in terminal cancer are little more than myth, handed down from one medical generation to the next. It is my hope, therefore, that this article will go some way to raising the subject from the realm of folklore into that of scientific fact.

Acknowledgments

The author wishes to thank Elizabeth Spinks for collating much of the provisional data and the Sir Halley Stewart Trust which awarded him a research fellowship. The work was supported by a grant from the Department of Health and Social Security, London.

References

Beaver, W. T., S. L. Wallenstein, R. W. Houde. and A. Rogers. 1966. "A Comparison of the Analgesic Effects of Pentazocine and Morphine in Patients with Cancer." *Clinical Pharmacology and Therapeutics* 7:740.

Bunyard, P. 1971. "Intractable Pain: How Treatable Is It?" *World Medicine* 17 (December 1).
Eddy, N. B., L. E. Lee, and C. A. Harris. 1959. "The Rate of Development of Physical Dependence and Tolerance to Analgesic Drugs in Patients with Chronic Pain. 1. Comparison of Morphine Oxymorphone, and Anileridine." *Bulletin on Narcotics* 11:3.
Fraser, H. F., H. Isbell, and D. A. Van Horn, 1957. "Effects of Morphine as Compared with a Mixture of Morphine and Diaminophenylthiazole (Daptazole)." *Anesthesiology* 18:531.
Galasko, C. S. B. and J. I. Burn, 1971. "Hypercalcaemia in Patients with Advanced Mammary Carcinoma." *British Medical Journal* 3:573.
Lasagna, L., and H. K. Beecher. 1974. "The Optimal Dose of Morphine." *Journal of the American Medical Association* 156:230.
Lee, L. E. 1942. "Studies of Morphine, Codeine, and Their Derivations." *Journal of Pharmacology and Experimental Therapeutics* 75:161.
Milton, G. W. 1972. "The Care of the Dying." *Medical Journal of Australia* 2:177.
Moertal, C. G., D. L. Ahmann, W. F. Taylor, and N. Schwartau. 1972. "A Comparative Evaluation of Marketed Analgesic Drugs." *New England Journal of Medicine* 286:813.
Paddock, R., G. Beer, J. W. Bellville, B. J. Ciliberti, W. H. Forrest, and E. G. Miller, 1969. "Analgesic and Side Effects of Pentazocine and Morphine in a Large Population of Postoperative Patients." *Clinical Pharmacology and Therapeutics* 10:355.
Robbie, D. S., and J. Samarasinghe. 1973. "Comparison of Aspirin-Codeine and Paracetamol-Dextropropoxyphene Compound Tablets with Pentazocine in Relief of Cancer Pain." *Journal of International Medical Research* 1:246.
Twycross, R. G. 1972. "The Use of Diamorphine in the Management of Terminal Cancer." *Journal of Thanatology* 2:733.
World Health Organization. 1972. *Opiates and Their Alternatives for Pain and Cough Relief.* Technical Report Series 495.
——— 1969. Report 16. Technical Report Series 407.

12
CONTINUING AND TERMINAL CARE— OVERVIEW OF ANALGESIA (HISTORICAL AND CHRONOLOGICAL EVOLUTION, 1978)

ROBERT G. TWYCROSS

Editors' Note: Owing to intense interest and even confusion relating to the role of diamorphine in the management of advanced cancer pain, the importance of chronologically reviewing this therapeutic modality as utilized in Great Britain is of great relevance within the context of this book. This manuscript, the *third* in this series, was read in 1978 at The Foundation of Thanatology-sponsored Symposium, "Use of Psychopharmacological and Analgesic Agents in the Clinical and Psychosocial Care of the Dying Patient and the Bereaved." It is included to represent the state of the art at *that* time. It is *not* intended to represent the state of the art in 1985.

A recent report has emphasized that many patients dying of cancer do so only after weeks or months of uncontrolled pain. Parkes (1976) compared hospital-centered and home-centered terminal care by means of postbereavement visits to the surviving spouse and found that about 20 percent of the hospital patients died with their severe and mostly continuous pain unrelieved. A similar percentage experienced pain of comparable intensity before admission, which suggests that admission to a hospital did not lead to improved relief. Of those who died at home, 10 percent had severe pain preterminally, but terminally the proportion rose to almost half. In contrast, following admission to St. Christopher's Hospice—a unit specializing in symptom control in far-advanced cancer—the percentage of patients with severe pain fell from 36 to 8.

In the home-based patients, the main reason for poor pain control appeared to be a failure on the part of the general practitioner to ensure that regular doses of an appropriate analgesic were given in sufficient quantity to alleviate the pain. One man of 54 became totally demoralized and for several months spent much of the time crying. He was so frightened that he clung to his wife and became "hysterical" whenever she left the room. He received an injection each *week* and was not able to go into hospital, because there was no bed available. Similar accounts given by other respondents suggested that neurotic exaggeration was not the explanation. Several patients put up with their pain without complaint on the supposition that nothing could be done to relieve it or that their chances of recovery would be enhanced if they refrained from taking powerful analgesics. The medical profession has a lot to learn before it can confidently assure patients that severe pain in advanced cancer can be controlled. Reasons for inadequate relief are many, but more fundamental than the incorrect use of analgesics is the tendency for a doctor to cease to be systematic when confronted with a dying patient. Instead of carefully analyzing the cause(s) of the patient's pain(s), the doctor prescribes a fixed dose of a standard preparation or, worse, underrates the intensity of a patient's discomfort and does nothing.

Assessment

Pain may be limited to one site or be multifocal. Each site where pain is felt should be recorded. The use of a body image to record the site(s) of pain is a great help. It acts as a baseline for future reference, facilitates patient management in situations where several doctors are involved, and helps in the consideration of underlying mechanisms (figure 12.1). Descriptions of

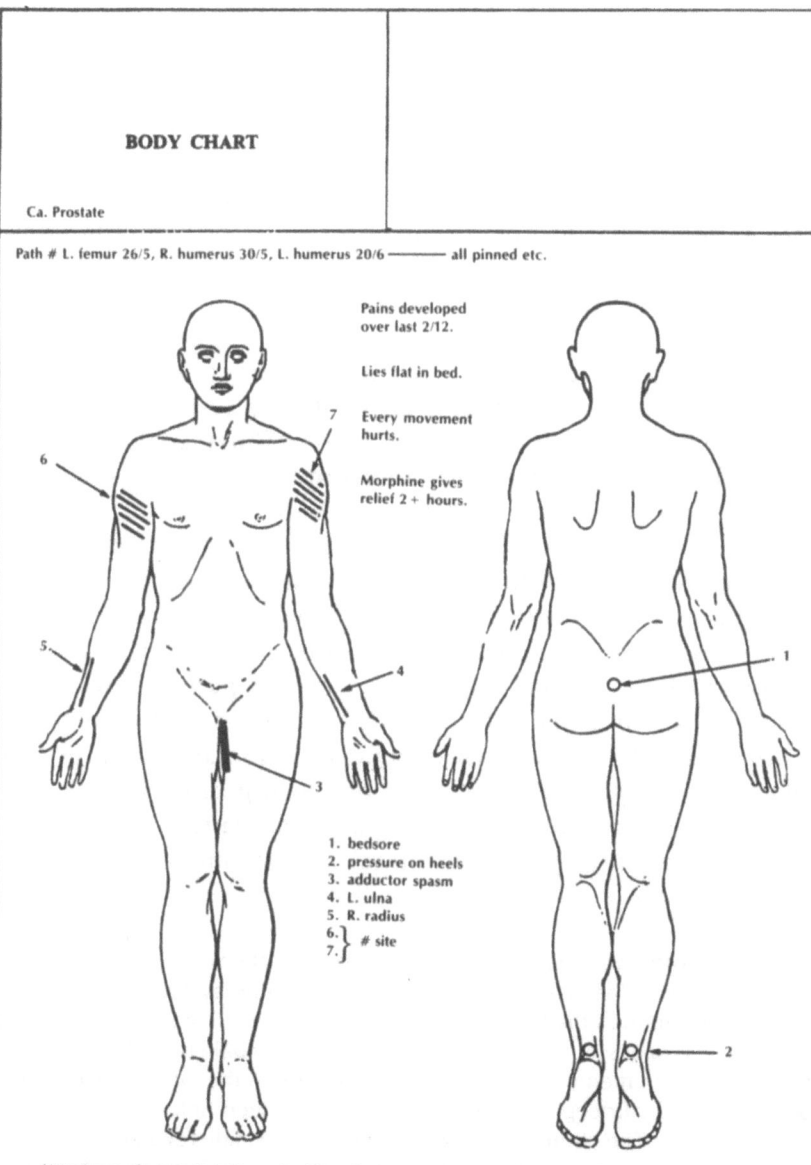

Figure 12.1. Pain chart of 65-year-old male with carcinoma of prostate. Adductor spasm is usually protective—that is, secondary to involvement of the pubis; treatment is as for bone pain, though sometimes diazepam may be necessary.

pain's being "like raving toothache" and "stabbing, especially when I move" point to nerve compression and influence the course of treatment if analgesics alone should fail to relieve (table 12.1). A diagnosis of cancer does not, however, mean that the malignant process is necessarily the cause of the pain. As in other areas of medicine, diagnosis must precede treatment. Bedsores, constipation, peptic ulcer, cystitis, or musculoskeletal disorders may prove to be the cause and are all conditions that benefit from specific treatment.

Intensity of pain is assessed not only by the patient's description but also by discovering what drugs have failed to relieve, whether sleep is disturbed, and in what way activity is limited ("How long is it since you went out?" "What are you doing around the house?" Etc.) In addition, the patient's spouse should be interviewed; generally speaking, one finds that patients have made light of their suffering. A patient may be in severe pain without looking distressed. With an obviously distressed patient who says or implies, "It's all pain, doctor," detailed assessment is impossible. In this situation the pain is compounded by anxiety and fear, and the patient should be reviewed after an initial injection of diazepam and diamorphine or morphine. The dose will depend on the patient's previous medication and general condition, but 10 mg of each is usually not excessive in a young or middle-aged patient.

In some patients, pain is minimal at rest but intolerable on movement.

> A four-year-old child with an inoperable pontine glioma experienced increasing pain in the head and occipital region. She lay flat all the time because elevation of the head caused a marked increase in pain. With this history it was necessary to postulate a local source of pain (possibly caused by postradiation meningeal adhesions) in addition to the diffuse headache of secondary hydrocephalus (which would have been helped by a more erect posture). The diffuse pain was relieved by small regular doses of morphine but not until she was transferred from a King's Fund to an Ellison bed (which elevates head, neck, and trunk in unison) was it possible for the child to sit up without pain. Subsequently, it became possible to transfer the child from bed to a high-backed reclining chair and, eventually, to lift her onto her mother's lap. This suggested that some of the pain had been caused by spasm of the neck muscles, and the confidence engen-

Table 12.1. Treatment of Pain in Advanced Cancer

Mechanism	Analgesic Adjuvants	Coanalgesic	Nondrug Treatment	Other Measures
1. Soft tissue infiltration				
2. Bone involvement		aspirin	radiotherapy	morphine (severe)
3. Nerve compression		prednisolone	nerve block*	— laxative
4. Raised cerebral pressure		dexamethasone		codeine (moderate)
5. Lymphodema		diuretic	compression sleeve	— anxiolytic?
6. Abdominal viceral a) epigastric b) hypogastric			celiac axis ganglion block (presacral block)*	aspirin (mild) antiemetic? modification of lifestyle diversion–heat–massage
7. Ulceration/infection		antibiotic		
8. Constipation	specific			
9. Second pathology	treatment			

*The use of nerve blocks for lower abdominal pain is limited by probability of causing urinary retention.

dered by the ability to sit up in bed allowed additional maneuvers to be undertaken without pain.

The probability of the initial prescription's being inadequate increases with the intensity of pain. Patients should, therefore, be reassessed within hours if the pain is overwhelming, or after one or two days if the pain is severe or moderate. If troublesome or unacceptable side effects result, treatment may need to be modified. In addition, the relief of the major pain may allow a second, less severe pain to become apparent.

> An 85-year-old man with carcinoma of the prostate and pain in the right femur caused by a metastasis was treated with aspirin and morphine. Casual questioning the next day indicated that although the pain was less severe, he was still in pain. Further questioning revealed that the site of pain was now retrosternal and epigastric; he had no femoral pain at all. The dose of morphine was, therefore, left unaltered, and the prescription of an antacid resulted in complete relief.

Pain Control

Relief of pain may be achieved by one or more of the following methods:

1. modification of pathological process
2. elevation of pain threshold
3. interruption of pain pathways
4. immobilization

Modification of Pathological Process

Osseous metastasis is the main cause of pain in the majority of patients with carcinoma of the breast, bronchus, or prostate. Bone pain is also common in carcinomata of the kidney and thyroid and in multiple myeloma. Modification of the pathology by radiation, chemotherapy, or hormone treatment should always be considered even in far-advanced cancer, though it is important to ensure that the treatment is not worse than the disease. Moreover, because androgens or estrogens have been prescribed, this does not mean that analgesics should be withheld. A combined approach should be employed. If relief is obtained and there are no complaints of "breakthrough" pain, then the analgesic regimen can be modified—a less potent analgesic can be prescribed or the treatment withdrawn completely.

Radiation therapy gives partial or even complete relief in 90 percent of patients experiencing bone pain, and generally may be administered in a single, nonfractionated dose. One study showed that although patients treated by single dose commonly had more nausea and vomiting, many of those receiving fractionated treatment were exhausted by the end of the course (Penn 1976). Fractionation is probably necessary only when there is a high risk of nausea and vomiting despite prophylactic antiemetics—for example, when irradiating in the region of L1 and when treating half or more of the pelvis.

Elevation of Pain Threshold

Pain is a dual phenomenon, one part being the perception of the sensation and the other the patient's emotional reaction to it. This means that attention must be paid to nondrug factors that modulate pain threshold, such as anxiety and depression, as well as to the correct use of analgesics and other drugs (table 12.2). Most patients fear the process of dying—"Will it hurt?" "Will I suffocate?"—and many fear death itself. Many of these fears remain unspoken unless the patient is given the opportunity to express them. Doctors need to give time and opportunity for patients to talk about their progress or lack of it. Tranquilizers have only a limited place in terminal cancer care. Patients who are markedly anxious or agitated usually need a combination of a tranquilizer and an analgesic; so does the patient with overwhelming pain.

Depression not only can, but frequently does, supervene in patients receiving so-called "euphoriant" drugs. The likelihood of this occurring increases the longer a patient is maintained on a narcotic analgesic (Twycross and Wald 1976). An antidepressant should be prescribed in these circumstances, starting with

Table 12.2. Factors Affecting Pain Threshold

discomfort		relief of symptoms
insomnia		sleep
fatigue		rest
anxiety	threshold	sympathy
fear	lowered	understanding
anger		diversion
sadness		elevation of mood
depression		
mental isolation		analgesics
introversion		tranquilizers	threshold raised
(past experience)		antidepressives

half the usual adult dose, for debilitated patients often become confused if a higher dose is given, particularly when other psychoactive drugs are being taken concurrently. Support and companionship are always necessary, particularly in cases where the depression is more properly described as sadness at the thought of leaving behind one's family, one's friends, and all that is familiar.

The use of analgesics is best seen as but one way—generally a powerful way—of elevating the pain threshold though a failure to allow patients to express their fears and anxieties can cause otherwise relievable pain to remain intractable.

Use of Analgesics

To allow pain to reemerge before administering the next dose not only causes unnecessary suffering but encourages tolerance. "Four-hourly as required" has no place in the treatment of persistent pain; whatever its etiology, *continuous pain requires regular preventive therapy*. The aim is to titrate the dose of the analgesic against the patient's pain, gradually increasing the dose until the patient is pain-free. The next dose is given before the effect of the previous one has worn off and, therefore, before the patient may think it necessary. In this way it is possible to erase the memory and fear of pain. Because patients do not like constantly taking tablets or receiving injections, a four-hourly interval between doses should be regarded as the norm, though sometimes more frequent administration may be necessary. Many patients do not require a dose in the middle of the night—though, if necessary, a patient should be wakened to take it (or set his alarm) rather than let him wake later complaining of pain.

The effective analgesic dose varies considerably from patient to patient; the right dose of any analgesic is that which gives adequate relief for at least three, preferably four or more hours. "Maximum" or "recommended" doses, derived mainly from postoperative parenteral single-dose studies, are not applicable in advanced cancer. For example, the effective dose of *oral* morphine ranges from as little as 5 mg to more than 100 mg every four hours. Patients will usually accept two, sometimes three, analgesic tablets per administration, together with additional medication; four or more tablets of the same preparation are not often acceptable. Generally, if two tablets are not adequate, the patient should be transferred to a more potent alternative. Pain unrelieved by other measures, not short life expectancy, is the primary criterion for prescription of morphine or other narcotic analgesics.

Antiinflammatory Drugs

The importance of aspirin in the relief of bone pain has been reemphasized (Twycross 1978). Many osseous metastases produce or induce the production of a prostaglandin (PG), probably PGE_2, which causes osteolysis (*Lancet* 1976) and also lowers the "peripheral pain threshold" by sensitizing free nerve endings (Ferreira 1972). Aspirin (in high dosage) and other nonsteroidal antiinflammatory drugs (NSAID) inhibit the synthesis of PGs and by so doing alleviate pain. This suggests that, compared with morphine, NSAID should be relatively more efficacious in bone pain than in pain caused by soft-tissue infiltration. Our experience in Oxford would support such a hypothesis (figure 12.2).

Response to PG inhibitors is, however, variable, a fact that can be explained if certain cancer cell types synthesize osteolytic agents other than or in addition to PGE_2. It has been shown, for example, in patients with hypercalcemia in association with multiple myeloma or a reticulosis, that the urinary excretion of PG metabolites is normal and that bone resorption appears to be due to secretion of "osteoclast activating factor" by tumor cells (Mundy et al. 1974). Other candidates include ectopic parathyroid hormone and active vitamin D metabolites or related sterols.

Despite the variable response it should not be regarded as a general rule that aspirin and other potent NSAID should be used either alone or in combination with a narcotic analgesic when one is seeking to relieve bone pain by pharmacologic means. Aspirin in a dose of between 3 and 6 grams a day has much to commend it and is available in a variety of preparations. Phenylbutazone commonly causes fluid retention, and in the elderly and debilitated, indomethacin is prone to cause or exacerbate neuropsychiatric disturbances. Newer agents such as flurbiprofen and diflunisal appear promising, and it is possible that they may prove useful in patients who fail to respond to aspirin.

Corticosteroids

Corticosteroids prevent the release of PGs by exerting a "stabilizing" affect on cell membranes; they do not inhibit PG synthesis. They do, however, have an impact on elements of the inflammatory process not connected with PGs and commonly stimulate appetite and elevate mood (*Drug Therapy Bulletin* 1974). Even so, clinical impression suggests that corticosteroids are not as effective as aspirin in relieving bone pain, though they are probably more effective in alleviating pain associated with extensive soft-tissue infiltration in relatively circumscribed areas—for example, head and neck cancers, or pelvic malignancy, and massive hepatic metastases. Sometimes, particularly with pelvic malignancy, greater relief is obtained by using both aspirin and prednisolone in association with a narcotic analgesic.

The usual starting dose is prednisolone 10 mg tid, reducing to 10 mg bid or 5 mg tid after a week. Prednisolone should also be used when pain is caused by nerve compression (*vide infra*). With headache caused by raised intracranial pressure, the more potent dexamethasone is often necessary, together with an analgesic. The usual starting dose is 4 mg tid, reducing, if possible, to 2 mg tid or less when the headache has been controlled satisfactorily.

Narcotic Analgesics

When the nonnarcotic analgesics (aspirin and paracetamol/acetominophen) fail to relieve, a weak narcotic such as codeine or dihydrocodeine should be prescribed alone or with aspirin or

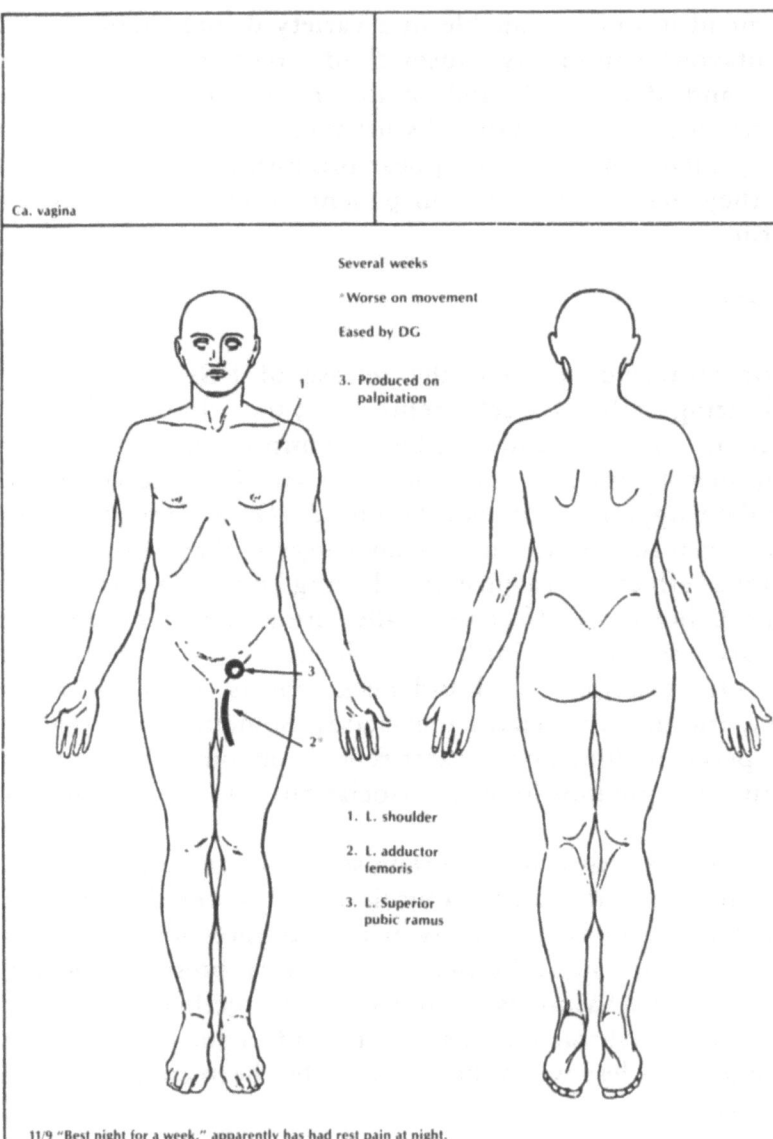

Figure 12.2. Pain charts of two patients with bone pain. Complete relief was obtained by using morphine and aspirin. In both, morphine was subsequently stopped without a return of pain, though after several weeks it became neces-

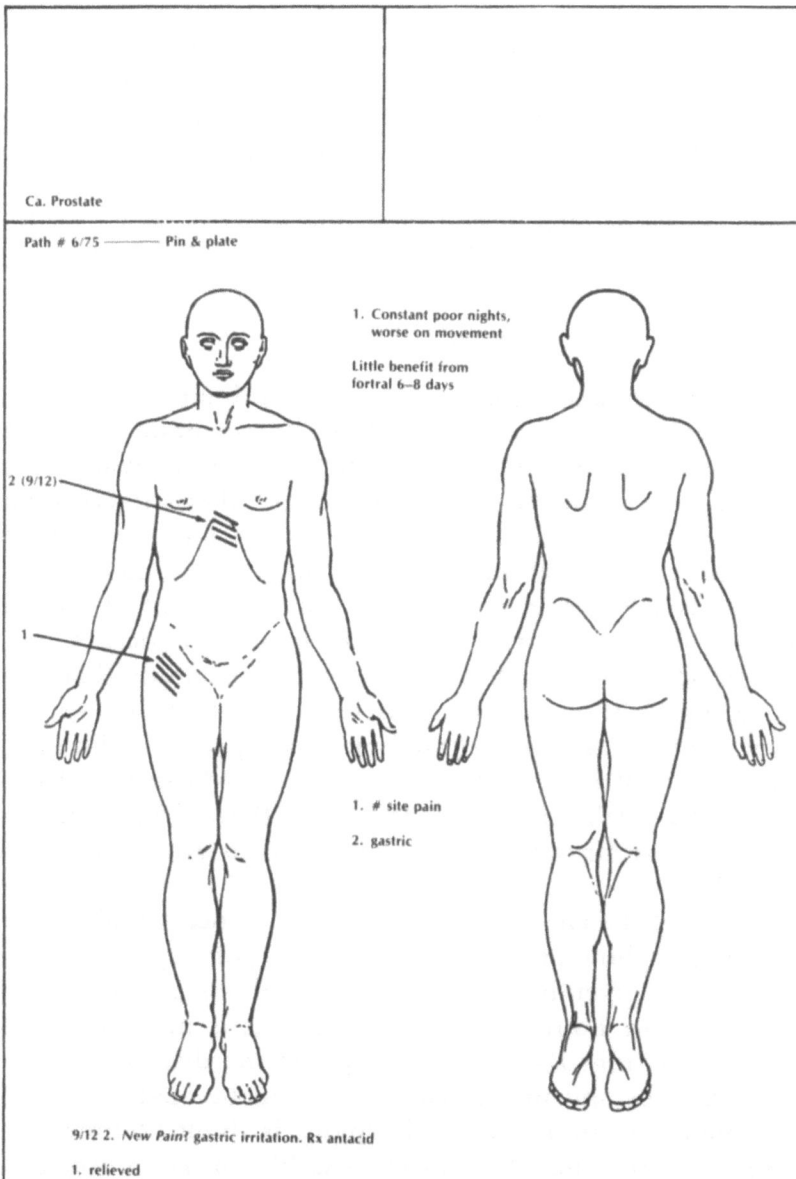

sary to represcribe it. Virtually bedfast when admitted, the patients charted in both 12.2a and 12.2b became fully mobile.

paracetamol. Pentazocine, a partial agonist, has no place in the treatment of cancer pain. By mouth it is not a potent analgesic; 50 mg of pentazocine is less effective than two tablets of aspirin-codeine, or paracetamol-propoxyphene (Robbie and Samarasinghe 1973). Moreover, the proportion of patients experiencing psychotomimetic side effects is unacceptably high, and although such side effects tend to be dose-related, they have been observed after even small doses by mouth. Similarly, orally administered pethidine/meperidine should not be regarded as a potent analgesic, and by injection it acts only for some two to three hours.

Papaveretum and dipipanone are useful intermediates between weak narcotics and morphine. Dipipanone is available only with cyclizine as Diconal, though there is no evidence that it causes more nausea than other narcotics. Alternatively, aspirin and opium (Nepenthe) may be used; each 1 ml of undiluted Nepenthe contains about 10 mg of morphine and is usually supplied as a 10 percent (1 ml in 10) or 20 percent (2 ml in 10) solution in chloroform water. Precipitation occurs when stronger solutions are dispensed. Dextromoramide (Palfium 5 and 10 mg), although potent, is relatively short-acting; it is, however, useful as "top up" medication for patients who experience occasional exacerbations of pain but whose pain for the most part is well controlled. (Some of these drugs, although used in Great Britain, are not available to American practitioners.)

The top of the analgesic ladder is not reached simply by prescribing morphine or diamorphine (diacetyl morphine, heroin). Both may be given in a wide range of oral doses, from 5 to 100 mg every four hours—though, in fact, it is unusual to need more than 30 mg. By mouth, morphine and dismorphine have similar actions and unwanted effects, but because of its more complete absorption, oral diamorphine is about 1½ times more potent than oral morphine (Twycross 1977b). Both opiates are commonly dispensed with cocaine in a vehicle containing alcohol and syrup ("the Brompton Cocktail"). Some patients, however, complain about the "sickliness" of such mixtures, while others dislike the alcoholic "bite." Moreover, the benefit of a small fixed dose of cocaine is probably slight and has, on occasion, caused restlessness and hallucinations in the elderly. It is my practice, despite the recent inclusion of a convenient formulation in the British National Formulary, to dispense morphine in chloroform water alone, the patient adding blackcurrent juice or other flavoring as desired. If dispensed in combination with prochlorperazine or chlorpromazine, the incorporation of one of the flavored proprietary syrups usually circumvents the need for additional flavoring.

When regular injections are required, I use diamorphine hydrochloride, available in ampoules as freeze-dried pellets. It is considerably more soluble than morphine sulfate—100 mg will dissolve in 0.2 ml. This means that the volume injected need never be large, an important consideration when repeated injections have to be given to a cachectic patient (table 12.3). Most patients can be maintained on oral medication. The main indication for parenteral administration, apart from the last few hours of life, is intractable nausea and vomiting despite the prescription of an antiemetic.

The need for injections may sometimes be avoided by using morphine suppositories. Several strengths are available, ranging from 10 to 60 mg. Proladone suppositories, which contain 30 mg of oxycodone pectinate, are also available; after administration the oxycodone is slowly released from the pectin core over several hours. Thus one or two suppositories every six or eight hours may be adequate. Fifteen mg of oxycodone is equivalent to 10 mg of morphine. Alternatively, round-the-clock relief may be maintained by using Duromorph, a microcrystalline suspension of morphine, two or three times a day. It is available as an intramuscular preparation in capped vials, each containing 70.4 mg of morphine base in 1.1 ml (64 mg/ml). The dose will depend on the patient's previous medication. For example, if one assumes a 1:3 oral to parenteral potency ratio for morphine, 32 mg of Duromorph (0.5 ml) b.d. will probably substitute adequately for 30 mg of oral morphine four-hourly.

Levorphanol (Dromoran 1.5 mg) and phenazocine (Narphen 5 mg) should be regarded as alternatives to morphine and diamorphine (table 12.4). By mouth on a weight-for-weight basis,

Table 12.3. Injection Volume of Equianalgesic Doses of Diamorphine and Morphine

Preparation	Solubility in water at 25°C (1G in x ml)	Potency Relative to Diamorphine	Available Ampules (mg/ml)	Volume of equianalgesic Doses (ml)			
				30	60	90	120mg
Diamorphine hydrochloride	1.6	1	(Freeze-dried)	0.1	0.1	0.15	0.2
			15*	4.0	4.0	12.0	16.0
Morphine sulfate	21	½	30†	2.0	4.0	6.0	8.0

*Maximum strength available in the United States.
†Maximum strength available in the United Kingdom.

Table 12.4. Approximate Oral Analgesic Equivalence of Potent Narcotics

Analgesic	Tablet	Dose of Diamorphine Hydrochloride	Dose of Morphine Sulfate
Dipipanone (Diconal)	10 mg (+ 30 mg cyclizine)	3 mg	5 mg
Papaveretum (Omnopon)	10 mg	3 mg	5 mg
Levorphanol (Dromoran)*	1.5 mg	5 mg	8 mg
Phenazocine† (Narphen)	5 mg	15 mg	25 mg
Nepenthe (undiluted)	1 mg	8 mg	12 mg

Note: *Dextromoramide* (Palfium). A single 5-mg dose is equivalent to diamorphine 10 mg/morphine 15 mg in terms of peak effect but acts only for 1–2 hours. Useful as an additional "as required" analgesic for intermittent, severe breakthrough pain.
*Methadone (Physeptone). A single 5-mg dose is equivalent ot diamorphine 5 mg/morphine 7.5 mg. Has a prolonged plasma half-time, which leads to *accumulation* when given repeatedly. Thus, it is several times more potent when given *regularly*.
†Often satisfactory 6-hourly.

both are approximately four to five times more potent than morphine and have a longer duration of action. Methadone (Physeptone) may also be useful in these circumstances but, because of its prolonged plasma half-time (Verebely et al. 1975), should be used with care, if at all, in the elderly or extremely debilitated.

Adjuvant Medication

Most patients with terminal cancer have more than one symptom. Nausea and vomiting are both common, and the use of a narcotic analgesic tends to precipitate or exacerbate these symptoms, particularly if the patient is ambulant. Patients prescribed a narcotic analgesic should be questioned about nausea and vomiting and either have an antiemetic (for example, prochlorperazine, metoclopramide, cyclizine) prescribed simultaneously or have the need for one reviewed two or three days later. Constipation almost always occurs when a narcotic is taken regularly but generally responds to the *regular* use of an appropriate aperient.

The value of diversional activity should not be forgotten. It ranges from backrubs to craft work, talking books, access to radio and television, someone to talk to, and dayroom activities. Pain is worse when it occupies the patient's whole attention. Diversional activity does much more than just "pass the time"; it also diminishes the pain.

Addiction

Although the term *drug addiction* has been replaced officially by *drug dependence,* unofficially it continues to be used. Drug dependence has been defined as:

> A state, psychic and sometimes also physical, resulting from the interaction between a living organism and a drug, characterized by behavioral and other responses that always include a compulsion to take the drug on a continuous or periodic basis in order to experience its psychic effects, and sometimes to avoid the discomfort of its absence. Tolerance may or may not be present [WHO 1969].

This is a broader definition than that of 1964, which emphasized the need for both tolerance and an early development of physical dependence in addition to strong psychological dependence (WHO 1964). The term *drug dependence* now more closely approximates to the popular conception of addiction—a compulsion or overpowering drive to take the drug in order to experience its psychological effects. Occasionally, a patient is admitted who appears to be addicted, demanding "an injection" every two or three hours. Typically such a patient has a long history of poor pain control and will for several weeks have been receiving fairly regular (four-hourly as required) but inadequate injections of one or more narcotic analgesics. Given time, it is usually possible to control the pain adequately, prevent clock watching and demanding behavior, and sometimes transfer the patient to an oral preparation. But even here, it cannot be said that the patient is addicted, because the patient is not demanding the narcotic in order to experience its psychological effect but to be relieved from pain for at least an hour or two.

Even so, many physicians are reluctant to use narcotic analgesics, particularly diamorphine or morphine, because they assume that tolerance will result in the medication's becoming ineffective. This is understandable, because little information has been available concerning the long-term effects of narcotic analgesics when administered regularly to relieve persistent pain. The lack of data resulted in predictions' being made on the basis of animal and human volunteer studies. However, in the studies using ex-addicts at the Addiction Research Center in Lexington, the emphasis has been on *inducing* tolerance and physical dependence as rapidly as possible by using maximum tolerated doses rather than on administering the drugs in doses and at intervals comparable to a clinical regimen (Isbell 1948). Although such studies have been useful in predicting abuse liability, their relevance to clinical practice is questionable.

To allow predictions to be made on the basis of clinical experience, the notes of 500 patients admitted consecutively to St. Christopher's Hospice were reviewed (Twycross 1974). Of these 500 patients, 218 received diamorphine regularly for at least one week. By grouping the patients according to survival after commencing diamorphine, it was demonstrated that *the longer the duration of treatment the slower the rate of rise in dose.* In a second review (Twycross and Wald 1976), 115 patients who had received diamorphine regularly for at least twelve weeks were selected from approximately 3,000 patients admitted over seven years. Dose-time charts were prepared. Visual analysis indicated that in many there was an initial phase when the dose was increased several times within one or two weeks followed by a prolonged phase when the dose was increased less often or not at all. It was also clearly demonstrated that *the longer a patient survived after prescription of diamorphine, the greater the likelihood of a reduction in dose.*

Dose reductions were made on a trial-and-error basis in patients who had improved generally over a number of weeks and who had had no recent episodes of "breakthrough" pain. Reductions were also made after successful intrathecal nerve blocks in five patients and after treatment with a cytotoxic agent or radiation in a number of others. A total of nine patients stopped receiving diamorphine; three stopped taking diamorphine altogether; four patients stopped for more than four months; and two stopped for approximately three weeks.

It was concluded that diamorphine, when used as part of a pattern of total care, may be used for long periods without concern about tolerance. Moreover, although physical dependence probably develops in most patients after several weeks of continuous treatment, this does not prevent the downward adjustment of dose when considered clinically feasible. Experience with methadone, levorphanol, and phenazocine suggests that the "natural history" of their long-term use in patients in pain is similar to that of diamorphine and morphine.

Interruption of Pain Pathways

Note, analgesics alone are often effective in relieving pain due to nerve compression. If the response is poor, however, the use of prednisolone 5–10 mg three times a day is recommended. By reducing inflammatory swelling around the growth, the effective tumor mass is reduced and the compression alleviated. In patients with a prognosis of only a few weeks, this may be sufficient to circumvent the need for chemical neurolysis. In those with a longer life expectancy, the pain may return as the tumor continue to grow; in these a nerve block will be required. In patients whose morale is low or precarious, it is advisable to warn that a block may become necessary in order to avoid loss of confidence if the pain should return.

Modification of Lifestyle

Some patients continue to experience pain on movement despite analgesics, other drugs, radiotherapy, and nerve blocks. In these, the situation may be improved by suggesting commonsense modifications to daily activity. For example, a man may continue to struggle to stand when shaving unless the doctor suggests that sitting would be a good idea. Such a suggestion is accepted more readily if accompanied by a simple explanation of why weightbearing precipitates or exacerbates the pain. Individually designed plaster or plastic supports for patients with multiple collapsed vertebrae or Thomas splints for femoral pain are occasionally necessary to overcome intolerable pain on movement in bedfast patients.

Internal fixation or the insertion of a prosthesis should be considered if a pathological fracture of a long bone occurs, because these measures obviate the need for prolonged bedrest, and pain is usually relieved. The decision whether or not to treat surgically depends on the patient's general condition, but whereas in bronchial carcinoma or malignant melanoma pathological fracture often presages death, in breast cancer this is not generally so, particularly if the tumor is hormone-sensitive. The median survival after the first or only pathological fracture associated with breast cancer is about six months, ranging from two months to four years (Twycross 1972).

Expectations

A survey of patients with persistent pain suggested that patient's expectations in relation to relief are lower than they need to be (Hunt et al. 1977). However, whereas relief is obtained within two or three days in some patients, in others, particularly those whose pain is made worse by movement and in the very anxious and depressed, it may take three or four weeks of treatment to achieve satisfactory control. Even so, it should be possible to achieve some improvement within 24 to 48 hours in all patients. Although the ultimate aim is complete freedom from pain, we will be less disappointed but, paradoxically, more successful if in practice we aim at "graded relief." Further, as some pains respond more readily than others, improvement should be assessed in relation to each pain.

The initial target should be a pain-free, sleepful night. Many patients have not had a good night's rest for weeks or months and are exhausted and demoralized. To sleep through the night pain-free and wake refreshed is a boost to both the doctor's and the patient's morale. Next, one aims for relief at rest in bed or chair during the day; finally, for freedom from pain on movement. The former is always eventually possible; the latter is not.

However, the encouragement that relief at night and when resting during the day brings gives patients new hope and incentive and enables them to begin to live again despite limited mobility. Freed from the nightmare of constant pain, their last weeks or months take on a new look.

The doctor must be determined to succeed and be prepared to spend much time assessing and reassessing the patient's pain and other symptoms. Decisive action is needed to avoid the reported situation of a ninety-year-old man, admitted to a London teaching hospital with bone pain, who died still in pain three months later (Hunt et al. 1977). With cancer one is dealing with a progressive pathological process This means that new pains may develop or old pains reemerge. It should not be assumed that a fresh complaint of pain merely calls for an increase in a previously satisfactory analgesic regimen; it demands reassessment, an explanation to the patient, and only then, modification of drug therapy or other intervention.

Acknowledgments.

Tables 12.1 and 12.4 and figures 12.1 and 12.2 are reproduced by permission of Pitman Medical, Tunbridge Wells, England.

References

"Corticosteroids in Terminal Cancer." 1974. *Drug Therapy Bulletin* 12:63–64.
Ferreira, S. H. 1972. "Prostaglandins, Aspirin-like Drugs, and Analgesia." *Nature and New Biology* 240:200–3.
Hunt, J. M., T. D. Stollar, D. W. Littlejohns, R. G. Twycross, and D. W. Vere. 1977. "Patients with Protracted Pain." *Journal of Medical Ethics* 3:61–73.
Isbell, H. 1948. "Methods and Results of Studying Experimental Human Addiction to Newer Synthetic Analgesics." *Annals of the New York Academy of Sciences* 51:108–22.
Mundy, G. R., L. G. Raisz, R. A. Cooper, G. P. Schechter, and S. E. Salmon. 1974. "Evidence for the Secretion of an Osteoclast Stimulating Factor in Myeloma." *New England Journal of Medicine* 291:1041–46.
"Osteolytic Metastases." 1976. *Lancet* 2:1063–64.
Parkes, C. M. 1976. "Home or Hospital?: Terminal Care as Seen by Surviving Spouses." *Journal of the Royal College of General Practice* 28:19–30.

Penn, C. R. H. 1976. "Single Dose and Fractionated Palliative Irradiation for Osseous Metastases." *Clinical Radiology* 27:405–8.
Robbie, D. S. and J. Samarasinghe. 1973. "Comparison of Aspirin-Codeine and Paracetamol-Dextropropoxyphene Compound Tablets with Pentazocine in Relief of Cancer Pain." *Journal of Internal Medical Research* 1:246–52.
Twycross, R. G. 1974. "Clinical Experience with Diamorphine in Advanced Malignant Disease." *International Journal of Clinical Pharmacology* 9:184–98.
―――― 1977a. "Care of the Terminal Patient." In B. A. Stoll, ed., *Breast Cancer Management: Early and Late*. London: Heinemann.
―――― 1977b. "Choice of Strong Analgesic in Terminal Cancer: Diamorphine or Morphine?" *Pain* 3:93–104.
―――― 1978. "Bone Pain in Advanced Cancer." In D. W. Vere, ed., *Topics in Therapeutics 4*. Tunbridge Wells: Pitman Medical.
Twycross, R. G. and S. J. Wald. 1976. "Long-Term Use of Diamorphine in Advanced Cancer." In J. J. Bonica and Albe-Fessard, eds., *Advances in Pain Research and Therapy*, vol. 1. New York: Raven Press.
Verebely, K., J. Volavka, S. Mule, and R. Resnick. 1975. "Methadone in Man: Pharmacokinetics and Excretion Studies in Acute and Chronic Treatment." *Clinical Pharmacology and Therapeutics* 18:180–90.
World Health Organization. Expert Committee on Drug Dependence. 1964. Report 13. Technical Report Series 287.
―――― 1969. Report 16. Technical Report Series 407.

13.
CANCER PAIN: A COMPARISON OF METHADONE, METHADONE-COCAINE, AND METHADONE-AMPHETAMINE

Michael Weintraub, Amy Valentine, and Steven Steckel

In 1896 Herbert Snow, writing in the *British Medical Journal*, told of his use of cocaine in conjunction with opium: "Over and above its value in sustaining vitality, the local anesthetic properties of cocaine are of great service in epithelioma of the tongue or mouth, as in gastric, intestinal or uterine lesions is its property of precluding emesis" (Snow 1896).

Some years later, chest surgeons at the Brompton's Hospital popularized an analgesic cocktail containing heroin, cocaine, alcohol, and flavoring. Their intention, it seems, was to counteract the respiratory repression of the narcotic with the central nervous system stimulant cocaine (Martindale 1977).

Several versions of combination analgesics continued to be used in the United Kingdom and elsewhere. However, a recent surge of interest has occurred on both sides of the Atlantic. Much of this relates to the hospice movement and to an individual, Dr. Robert Twycross, whose work stimulated this research project and those of others.

This project began following a conference I (M.W.) conducted on pain control in cancer patients. I had mentioned that

Twycross' work (1974) as well as a paper by Forrest and others (1973), presented at the American Society for Clinical Pharmacology and Therapeutics meetings, supported the hypothesis that central nervous system (CNS) stimulants potentiate narcotic analgesics. A nurse, Amy Valentine, who had become interested in the use of these combinations, had the formula for a "Brompton's" cocktail used in another institution. Later that afternoon, she called me to discuss the use of that recipe on a patient in the oncology clinic. We met with Steve Steckel, a pharmacist with a special interest in oncology. The idea of using diethyl morphine, the narcotic in the formula in question, did not, however, appear logical to me. Methadone, with its longer half-life, better oral/parenteral ratio, pharmaceutic stability, and ease of making up into a liquid formulation (elixir), seemed a more likely candidate for our version of Brompton's cocktail.

After our success with the first patient, we decided to test several cocktail mixtures to see if there really was an advantage, either increased efficacy or decreased toxicity, to adding CNS stimulants to methadone alone; to see if cocaine differed from amphetamine as the stimulant; and to see what happened to the analgesic response over one week.

This discussion presents our study design and methods, results, and conclusions drawn from the outcome of the study.

Methods

Medications

The three formulas were made up in 99 percent ethanol with a standard flavoring syrup (peppermint-raspberry). Each contained 1 mg of methadone syrup per ml of elixir. The cocaine concentration was 1 mg/ml and the amphetamine, 0.5 mg/ml of the d,1 racemate. The starting dose was 10 ml every 4 hours around the clock.

Patients

To enter the study, patients had to have moderate or severe pain despite an adequate trial (in both dose and duration) of narcotic analgesic therapy excluding methadone. All other treatment for the primary disease or the painful process, such as radiation therapy for bony metastases or antibiotics and drainage of abscesses, should have been undertaken. Current medications—for example, antinausea medications, psychotropics, and antibiotics—were continued throughout the study period. They could be changed as needed by the physicians in charge of the patient's care.

Study Design

We elected to do a double-blind comparison of the three formulas. Each patient received only one treatment, methadone (M), methadone plus cocaine (M-C), or methadone plus amphetamine (M-A). Patients and their physicians could increase or decrease the dose as needed to achieve maximum pain relief or diminish undesirable effects. The treatment assignment, while randomized, was stratified according to initial pain severity. We hoped in this way to avoid a preponderance of patients with severe or moderate pain in any group.

Assessment of Response

Since one of the goals of this study was to assess the efficacy of multiple doses of the formulas, we interviewed the patients 24 hours, 48 hours, and one week after starting treatment. A modification of the standard University of Rochester analgesic efficacy questionnaire (table 13.1) was used to collect the data. The interviewer was not aware of which treatment any patient received. Data on pain severity, pain relief, undesirable effects of the drugs, and effects on appetite and sleep were collected. The patient's dose of elixir was also noted. Finally, the observer

Table 13.1. University of Rochester Pain Study Questionnaire, modified by including dose, appetite, and sleep effects and changing time of assessment.

Patient Number/Drug Number	Severity of Pain	Baseline	24 Hours	48 Hours	1 Week
Patient's name	¹None				
History number	Slight or mild				
Date of attack	Moderate				
Age/sex	Severe				
Weight/Height	Very Severe				
Time of administration	²Completely gone				
Concomitant medication	> Half gone				
	< Half gone				
	Unchanged				
	Increased				
Food Intake	Pain location				
Appetite:	Pain quality				
Good	Temperature				
Fair	Blood pressure:				
Poor	Supine				
	Sitting				
Other effects	Interviewer				
Overall assessment	Side effects				
Compared to usual therapy	Scale score				

Side effects:
1. Nausea
2. Vomiting
3. Vertigo
4. Headache
5. Lightheadedness
6. Drowsiness
7. Pruritus
8. Dry mouth

Pain Quality:
1. Dull
2. Sharp

A. Steady
B. Throbbing

made a judgment on how well the medication worked. This integrated analgesia, the patient's activity level compared to baseline, and adverse effects for a global evaluation of the drug.

The measurements reported here are (1) pain relief score, where 0 stands for absence of pain and 4 stands for an increase in pain; (2) the number of patients in each pain relief class at the end of one week of treatment; (3) the severity of pain, where 0 is no pain and 4 is very severe pain; (4) the observer evaluation; (5) the mean dose of medication used by each treatment group, and (6) adverse effects.

A standard pain study convention was used, where noted, to compensate for missing data. The score on the previous assessment replaced the missing value. This system tends to magnify differences between drugs when the missing data come from patients who dropped out of the study because of medication failure.

Results

Patient Characteristics (tables 13.2–4).

Thirty-four patients participated in the study. There was a higher proportion of women in the M-A group—66 percent versus 50 percent in the methadone and M-C groups. The M-A group was younger on average and more of them took Di-

Table 13.2. Patients Characteristics: Methadone Group

Patient*	Age/Sex	Previous Medication
4M	58/M	Demerol, 75 mg q3 po
5M	42/M	Demerol, 100 mg q4 po
6M	45/M	Dilaudid, 4 mg q4 po
		Percodan, 2 mg q4 po
12M	55/F	Percodan, 2 mg q4 po
3S	57F	Morphine, 15 mg q3 sc
5S	32/M	Demerol, 125 mg q3 po
10S	70/F	Demerol, 50 mg q4 po
11S	65/M	Demerol, 150 mg q3 iv
12S	43/F	Dilaudid, 3 mg q3h
16S	57/F	Percodan, 2 mg q2h
17S	57/F	Percodan, 2 mg q2h
21S	60/M	Dilaudid, 4 mg q4 po

*M indicates that the patient entered the study with moderate pain; S, with severe pain.

Table 13.3. Patient Characteristics: Methadone-Cocaine Group

Patient*	Age/Sex	Previous Medication
2M	70/F	Dilaudid, 4 mg q6h
3M	56/M	Morphine, 4 mg q6 iv
8M	61/M	Percodan, 1 mg q3
9M	54/F	Percodan, 1 mg q3
4S	70/M	Dilaudid, 3 mg q6
7S	59/M	Dilaudid, 2 mg q4
8S	51/F	Dilaudid, 4 mg q4h
		Numorphan, 5 mg bid
14S	61/F	Percodan, 1 mg q3h
15S	56/M	Percodan, 2 mg q4h
22S	62/F	Talwin, 50 mg q4h

*M = moderate pain; S = severe pain (see table 1).

Table 13.4. Patient Characteristics: Methadone-Amphetamine Group

Patient*	Age/Sex	Previous Medication
1M	24/F	Not recorded
7M	47/F	Dilaudid, 2 mg q4h
10M	51/F	Morphine, 4 mg q4h iv
		Numorphan, 5 mg q4
11M	57/F	Dilaudid, 4 mg q4h
13M	51/M	Tylenol/codeine, 2 mg q2h
1S	41/M	Percodan, 2 mg q4h
		Dilaudid, 2 mg q4h
2S	62/F	Dilaudid, 4 mg q8h
6S	52/F	Percodan, 2 mg q2h
9S	44/M	Dilaudid, 8 mg q4h
13S	54/F	Dilaudid, 2 mg q4h
18S	65/M	Dilaudid, 2 mg q3h
20S	48/F	Dilaudid, 6 mg q3h

*M = moderate pain; S = severe pain (see table 1).

laudid. The dose equivalents of narcotics were also higher in this group than in the M-C group but not higher than in the M group. None of these differences was statistically significant.

At the time of entry into the study, six patients in the M group and two each in the M-C and M-A groups were receiving phenothiazines or trimethobenzamine HCl (Tigan) for control of nausea.

Analgesic Efficacy

Methadone-amphetamine was the most active combination as measured by the patients' assessment of pain relief (table 13.5).

Table 13.5 Patients' Evaluation of Pain Relief*

Time on Study	Methadone	Methadone-Cocaine	Methadone-Amphetamine
24 hr	1.8 ± 1.3	1.8 ± 1.2	1.6 ± 1.3
48 hr	1.1 ± 1.0	1.6 ± 1.0	1.1 ± 1.0
1 week	1.3 ± 0.9	1.7 ± 1.4	0.7 ± 0.7
Adjusted score†	1.7 ± 0.2	1.7 ± 0.5	0.8 ± 0.2‡

*Pain relief was based on a scale of 0 (pain completely gone) to 4 (pain increased). Values are mean ± S.D.
†Calculated to compensate for missing data from dropouts at 48 hours and one week: methadone group, 4 dropouts; methadone-cocaine, 3; methadone-amphetamine, 1.
‡Significantly different from Methadone, $p < 0.05$.

Using the missing-data convention magnifies the difference between M-A and M. All the patients still in the study receiving M-A had 50 percent or more pain relief at the one-week assessment (table 13.6). Note that more patients stayed in the M-A group and that 9 of the 10 scores are in the best categories.

Also noted was a definite continued improvement in mean pain severity scores in the M-A patients during the one-week treatment period. These scores leveled off after twenty-four hours in the other two treatment groups. All three analgesics lowered pain from "severe" to just above "moderate" (M-C) or even just above "mild" (M-A).

The differences in pain relief or severity are not statistically significant, although the trend is in favor of M-A.

The investigator's ratings (table 13.7), made before the codes were broken, show that all three elixirs seemed to work but the M-A group contained no failures, again showing a trend in favor of that combination. This score includes an assessment of analgesia, activity level, and adverse effects.

Table 13.6 Patient Evaluation of Pain Relief One Week After Starting Study*

Pain Relief	Methadone	Methadone-Cocaine	Methadone-Amphetamine
100%	0	1	4
> 50%	4	3	5
< 50%	2	1	1
No change	0	1	0
Worse	0	1	0

*Patients still in study.

Cancer Pain

Table 13.7 Observer's Evaluation*

Evaluation	Methadone	Methadone-Cocaine	Methadone-Amphetamine
Excellent	0	2	1
Good	7	3	4
Fair	2	3	7
Poor	0	1	0
None	3	1	0

*The investigator was not aware of treatment.

Since dose titration was allowed to achieve the therapeutic goal, the mean daily dose of drug used is an important measure of effect (table 13.8). Patients were thus involved in their therapy to the extent that they could adjust the dose of drug. As expected, patients with moderate pain used less of each of the drugs than those with severe pain. However, a look at overall drug use in the three groups reveals that the better analgesic results were obtained with a lower dose of M-A than of M. There was little difference between M-A and M-C doses. Again, although the numerical difference is great between the mean daily dose of M and M-A (16.4 ml per day in the severe group and 9.4 ml in all patients), it is not statistically significant but represents 16 and 9 mg of methadone respectively. Mean drug doses decreased from the initial level (60 ml a day) for all groups except the M severe.

More patients dropped out from the M group than from the other groups (table 13.9, table 13.10).

The expected undesirable effects of narcotics occurred in all three groups, although fewer of the M-A patients had adverse gastrointestinal effects (nausea and vomiting or constipation). One or two patients in all treatment groups had hallucinations. On the other hand, sleeplessness and decreased appetite were

Table 13.8 Mean Daily Doses of Elixir*

Pain Study	Methadone	Methadone-Cocaine	Methadone-Amphetamine
Severe	64.2 ± 11.5 (7)†	45.5 ± 5.5 (6)	47.8 ± 12.4 (7)
Moderate	30.7 ± 5.7 (3)†	36.7 ± 12.0 (3)†	41.3 ± 9.4 (4)†
Combined	54.2 ± 9.5 (10)	42.5 ± 5.2 (9)	44.8 ± 8.3

*In ml on last day of treatment; mean ± S.D. for number of patients in parentheses.
†Data not available for one patient.

Table 13.9 Adverse Effects

Symptom	Methadone	Methadone-Cocaine	Methadone-Amphetamine
Nausea	2	3	1
Vomiting	2	1	0
Constipation	0	1	1
Drowsiness	0	3	3
Hallucinations	2	1	1
Tachycardia	0	0	1

not reported in either of the CNS-stimulant treated groups. In fact, on direct questioning, 8 of the 22 patients on M-C or M-A reported improved sleep or appetite, or both.

Tables 13.11–13 contain a summary of the dose of medication, adverse effects, and appropriate comments on each patient's course.

Discussion

All three treatments were effective analgesics in this difficult-to-treat population. In general, M-A was better than M and better than or equal to M-C by all of the measurements. Although none of the differences was statistically significant, the lower dose, decreased incidence of adverse effects, and fewer dropouts indicate that the better ratings by patients and observers for M-A are clinically significant. The dose of amphetamine was unfortunately lower than that originally intended. A higher dose might have potentiated the analgesic more, but it might have increased undesirable effects as well.

Table 13.10 Patients Not Completing Study

Reason for Withdrawal	Methadone	Methadone-Cocaine	Methadone-Amphetamine
Adverse effects			
Nausea, hallucinations	3	3	
Nausea			1
Disease progression	1		1
Total	4	3	2

Cancer Pain

Table 13.11 Dose and Drug Effects: Methadone Group

Patient*	Dose (ml)	Adverse Effects	Comment
4M	25	Slight nausea	Euphoria; "holds better"
5M	—	Vomiting	Refused drug; off study
6M	42		Sleep and appetite improved
12M	25		Appetite and sleep better
3S	105		? Less sedated
5S	80	Hallucinations	Off study
10S	40	Hallucinations	Off study
11S	90	Bowel obstruction, nausea	Off study
12S	75	Vomited	Sleep and appetite better
16S			Activity and sleep better
17S	30		
21S	30		

*M = moderate pain; S = severe pain (see table 1).

In view of the recent finding that the oral absorption of cocaine is greater than previously believed (Van Dyke et al. 1978), our suggestion to the patients to swish the medication around in the mouth may not have been necessary. These recent data on cocaine pharmacokinetics suggest that there was a large disparity between the dose of cocaine and the dose of amphetamine in terms of CNS stimulation.

The benefits that we hoped would result from using methadone in the combination were achieved. Most patients were able to decrease drug intake during the one-week test period, perhaps because of the body's accumulation of methadone, which has a long half-life. Parenteral narcotics were rarely

Table 13.12 Dose and Drug Effects: Methadone-Cocaine Group

Patient	Dose (ml)	Adverse Effects	Comment
2M	20	Sedation; constipated	Sleep better
3M			
8M	30	Drowsy	Sleep and appetite better
9M	60		Activity and sleep better
4S	30	Hallucinations	Off study
7S	45		Initially better sleep and appetite
8S	60	Drowsy; confused	Slept better
14S	48	Nausea; sedation	
15S	60	Nausea; vomiting	Off study
22S	30	Nausea	Off study

Table 13.13 Dose and Drug Effects: Methadone-Amphetamine Group

Patient	Dose (ml)	Adverse Effects	Comment
1M	15		
7M			? Compliance
10M	60		Disease progression
11M	45	Nausea	Off study
13M	45		Cord compression; off study
1S	20	Drowsiness	
2S	15	Hallucinations; excess sedation	Naloxone given and dose lowered
6S	90	Constipated	Slept well
9S	23		"Better than Dilaudid"; activity and appetite better
13S	30		Disease worse; hospitalized
18S	60		
20S	90	Tachycardia; sedation	Slept well

needed. The drug was easy for the patients to use and titrate. It did not cause intolerable sedation by itself.

The effect of adequate pain control evidently overcomes any undesirable CNS-stimulating or appetite-suppressant effects of the combinations tested. With good analgesia patients slept and ate better. Addition of CNS stimulants did not increase the incidence of hallucinations. Those that did occur may have been related to disease, pain, or narcotic analgesics. At the doses tested we did not find serious cardiovascular toxicity from the stimulants used in the combinations.

Because the number of patients was small and the number of variables in the study was large, we are not surprised that clear statistical superiority of one of the three active analgesics over the other two could not be shown. Imbalance related to treatment assignment, such as having younger patients concentrated in the M-A group, probably biased the study against this particular combination. Bellville et al. (1971) demonstrated that age was a very important factor determining a patient's response to potent analgesics. With increasing age his patients had an increased analgesic response to the same dose of morphine. Despite problems such as this, by many measurements—some of which are not covariates—M-A appears to be very effective in providing excellent analgesia with few adverse effects.

Amphetamine itself has mild analgesic properties, which are probably of little clinical significance at these doses. Many reports have, however, indicated that CNS stimulants potentiate narcotic analgesics (Ivy et al. 1944, Mount et al. 1976, Melzack et al. 1976, Forrest et al. 1977). No theoretical basis for the potentiation has been verified experimentally. CNS stimulants may act by increasing sensory inflow, which might be expected to diminish the influence of any one stimulus, such as pain. This would be the opposite of the apparent increase in pain that a patient feels just after getting into bed or at any time of quiet reponse when external sensory stimuli diminish. Both narcotics and CNS stimulants have been shown to alter CNS neurotransmitter (dopamine, norepinephrine) concentrations and kinetics. Stimulants may alter enkephalin (or endorphin) kinetics, affecting their synthesis, release, or degradation in a manner that would increase efficacy. Or the effect of these "endogenous opioids" may be enhanced via a receptor interaction mechanism rather than pharmacokinetically. Stimulants may affect the pharmacokinetics of narcotic analgesics in some subtle, unknown way that enhances analgesia.

Melzack and coworkers (1976) believe that the effectiveness of the narcotic-CNS stimulant combination relates to the gate control theory of pain and to the fact that they act on different aspects of the pain experience, such as perception of the stimulus, the evaluation of the stimulus, and its emotional effects. The environment in which the combination is administered also had an effect in their study. In a well-run palliative-care unit with special support (psychic and physical facilities), the analgesic response was enhanced. Our patients were generally in standard two-patient hospital rooms or with family at home. Nonetheless, good response was obtained.

We believe that the data presented here do not support the now fashionable practice of nearly exclusive use of narcotic-CNS stimulant combinations. Twycross (1977) has written that he no longer uses the combinations unless a test dose of amphetamine with diamorphine enhances analgesia over that achieved by narcotics alone. Only then does he prescribe a diamorphine (heroin)-cocaine mixture.

The practice of using combinations for all patients seems aimed at increasing efficacy and decreasing adverse effects. However, not every patient—terminally ill or not, (with cancer or not—needs the extra medication in the cocktails or even a narcotic analgesic. The clinical pharmacology group at the University of Rochester, headed by Dr. Louis Lasagna, has developed several approaches to "escalation" of pain medications in cancer patients. Depending on the clinical picture, nonsteroidal antiinflammatory agents, combinations of tricyclic antidepressants and phenothiazines, and intramuscular methotrimeprazine (given to produce a restful, pain-free period), used where indicated, often provide full analgesia and enable the patient to be as active as possible. We also stress that methadone given by itself remains a valuable analgesic.

Tolerance to the analgesic effects of methadone alone or in combination posed no great problem either in this study or in subsequent use, despite administration of the drugs around the clock. We found, as others have reported, that once analgesia was achieved with these mixtures, patients were able to decrease the dose and increase the interval between doses while maintaining pain relief and thus manifesting maintained effectiveness. The addition of CNS stimulants did not, in the short period of this study, seem to affect the development of tolerance to the analgesic effects of methadone.

Some physicians using combinations of narcotics and cocaine routinely give phenothiazines to their patients. We elected not to do so, since we wanted to see whether the combinations might cause less nausea than methadone alone. This did seem to be the case, at least for methadone-amphetamine, from which few patients had gastrointestinal undesirable effects, and few required phenothiazines to be added.

At Strong Memorial Hospital, (Rochester, NY) when patients need more analgesia than that provided by narcotics alone (plus nonsteroidal antiinflammatory agents or other analgesics), we now use the methadone-amphetamine mixture, 1 mg of each (using d-amphetamine) per ml of elixir. In addition to its greater efficacy and fewer adverse effects, fluctuation in the availability of cocaine is another reason for using M-A. We do, however, have difficulty in obtaining methadone syrup, because of restriction of its use to methadone maintenance clinics.

References

Bellville, J. W. and W. A. Forrest, E. Miller, and B. W. Brown. 1971. "Influence of Age on Pain Relief from Analgesics: A Study of Postoperative Patients." *Journal of the American Medical Association* 217:1835–41.

Forrest, W. H., C. R. Brown, D. C. Mahler, J. Katz, P. Schroff, R. DeFalque, B. Boon, and K. James. 1973. "The Evaluation of Morphine and Dextroamphetamine Combinations for Analgesia." *Clinical Pharmacology and Therapeutics* 14:132.

Forrest, W. H., W. B. Byron, C. R. Brown, R. DeFalque, M. Gold, H. E. Gordon, K. E. James, J. Katz, D. L. Mahler, F. Schroff, and G. Teutsch, 1977. "Dextroamphetamine with Morphine for the Treatment of Postoperative Pain." *New England Journal of Medicine* 296:712–15.

Ivy, A. C., F. R. Goetzl, and D. Y. Burril. 1944. "Morphine Dextro-Amphetamine Analgesia." *War Medicine* 6:67–71.

Martindale, 1977. *The Extra-Pharmacopoeia*. A. Wade, ed. 27th ed. London: Pharmaceutical Press, 973.

Melzack, R., J. G. Ofresh, and B. M. Mount. 1976. "The Brompton Mixture: Effects on Pain in Cancer Patients." *Canadian Medical Association Journal* 115:125–29.

Mount, B. M., I. Ajemian, and J. F. Scott. 1976. "Use of the Brompton Mixture in Treating the Chronic Pain of Malignant Disease." *Canadian Medical Association Journal* 115:122–24.

Snow, H. 1896. "Opium and Cocaine in the Treatment of Cancerous Disease." *British Medical Journal* 2:718–19.

Twycross, R. G. 1974. "Clinical Experience with Diamorphine in Advanced Malignant Disease." *International Journal of Clinical Pharmacology* 9:184–98.

———1977. "Value of Cocaine in Opiate-Containing Elixirs." *British Medical Journal* 2:1348.

Van Dyke, C. R. Jatlow, J. Ungerer, P. G. Barash, and R. Byck. 1978. "Oral Cocaine: Plasma Concentrations and Central Effects." *Science* 200:211–13.

14.
UTILITY OF A COMBINATION OF STIMULANT DRUGS WITH OPIATES IN THE PRODUCTION OF ANALGESIA

WAYNE O. EVANS

In the search for the perfect analgesic, it has often occurred to investigators that an improvement in the effect of opiates might be forthcoming if other drugs were mixed with them to overcome or antagonize some of their undesirable side effects. As early as 1944, Ivy and his colleagues demonstrated that amphetamine could potentiate opiate-induced analgesia in dogs, mice, and man. In man, 16 mg of morphine in combination with 20 mg of dextroamphetamine produced a degree of analgesia 60 percent greater than with the same dose of morphine alone. At the same time, this mixture of drugs overcame the depression induced by morphine on respiration and blood pressure, and it reduced nausea and vomiting.

Between 1944 and 1950, the potentiation of opiate analgesia by substances of the amphetamine class was confirmed by Nickerson and Goodman (1947) with normal human subjects using isonipecaine. In addition, Nickerson (1950), by testing the reduction of pain produced by a hand emerged in ice water, showed the opiate-potentiating effects of amphetamines. He used a combination of 100 mg of meperidine and 10 mg of dextroamphetamine.

The first large-scale clinical test of an opiate mixed with amphetamine was conducted in 1951 by Abel and his associates.

(Abel and Harris 1947; Abel et al. 1951). They demonstrated in 7000 obstetrical cases that adding 5 mg of dextroamphetamine to 10 mg of morphine would provide good analgesia with a minimum of side effects. They also found a shortening of the length of time to first inspiration of the newborn infant with this mixture as compared with the inspiration time for infants of patients given morphine alone.

Other investigators have demonstrated that drugs that deplete the central nervous sytem of biogenic amines could antagonize the effects of opiates. Takagi et al. (1964) demonstrated the antagonism of the analgesic effects of morphine on mice with tetrabenazine and reserpine. This demonstrated that the presence of the putative neurotransmitters of the alpha adrenergic nervous system was a requirement for an effective analgesia with opiates.

The first serious proposal for the development of a useful clinical mixture of alpha-adrenergic stimulants, such as amphetamine, with opiates for clinical use occurred in 1962 (Evans 1962). This call for a study of the clinical utility of the synergism between these substances led in 1964 to a demonstration that by combining amphetamine with morphine in normal human beings the depressing effects of the opiate upon human cognition could be reversed (Evans and Smith 1964). This was the first double-blind, controlled study of the substances in man. It explored the full range of operational categories of human cognition that were known at that time.

At approximately the same time, studies using the self-injection technique in monkeys demonstrated that the addiction potential of the combination of amphetamine with an opiate was no greater than for the opiate alone (Deneau 1970). Other tests in mice established that the LD_{50} for the combination of the stimulant with the opiate was no greater than for the opiate alone. From these animal tests it could be seen that such a combination did not increase the danger of the drugs.

In 1967 Evans reported the first double-blind, controlled study of the use of a combination of amphetamine and morphine in a clinical population. Subjects for the study were young males suffering postoperative pain due to a hernia operation.

The subjects were divided into four groups and assigned treatment with morphine sulfate alone at 10 mg, or dextroamphetamine alone at 10 mg, or a combination of 10 mg of morphine plus 10 mg of dextroamphetamine, or isotonic saline as a placebo. They were tested at 45 and 90 minutes after the administration of drugs. At the same time that the measurements of analgesia were made, vital signs were measured. The study found that the following percentages of subjects showed half or more reduction in pain: 40 percent of the subjects receiving placebo, 57 percent of those receiving morphine, 72 percent of those receiving dextroamphetamine, and 96 percent of those receiving the mixture. The expected depression of vital signs was shown for morphine alone, whereas both the dextroamphetamine alone and the mixture of morphine plus dextroamphetamine produced no depression of vital signs. Nausea was also reduced by the mixture. Reports from the staff of the hospital conducting the study stated that the patients on the mixture were alert, jovial, and happy. This alertness was regarded as a disadvantage of the mixture by some of the staff, particularly by those nurses who seemed to feel that a sedated patient was a good patient.

In 1970, Forrest et al. evaluated the analgesic effectiveness of 5- and 10-mg doses of morphine with and without the addition of 10 mg of dextroamphetamine and found the combination of morphine and dextroamphetamine to be 1.5 times as potent in relieving pain as morphine alone. These studies were carried out on postoperative patients in a Veterans Administration hospital.

In 1972, Jasinski and Nutt tested morphine, dextroamphetamine, and a mixture of morphine and dextroamphetamine in a group of former addicts using a double-blind design. The subjective effects were measured by using the Addiction Research Center Inventory. Physiological effects also observed were pupil size, pulse rate, rectal temperature, systolic and diastolic blood pressure, and respiration. The outcomes of these studies showed an antagonism of the morphine-induced depression of vital signs by dextroamphetamine. The addition of dextroamphetamine to the morphine added to the euphoria of the morphine but did not significantly enhance the "liking" scores. The combination produced little evidence of sedation.

Lehmann et al. (1971) tested a combination of meperidine and dextroamphetamine on a population of 22 psychiatric, depressed patients. The patients were given 10 mg of dextroamphetamine orally and 50 mg of meperidine intermuscularly on alternate days, three times a week during a two-week period. Statistically significant improvements were noted on the symptoms of depressed mood, early waking insomnia, work and activities, diurnal variation, feelings of helplessness, suicidal tendencies, and worthlessness. They noted that the treatment was effective in both the young and in the geriatric patients and in both acute and chronic patients. There was a slow and sustained improvement throughout treatment. They found minimal side effects.

In a double-blind, single-dose study, Forrest et al. (1977) reported a 450-patient postoperative study. Each patient received one treatment of morphine sulfate (3, 6, or 12 mg) with dextroamphetamine (0, 5, or 10 mg). Analgesia was measured by the patient's subjective response to questions about the relief of pain. The combination of dextroamphetamine (10 mg) with morphine was twice as potent as morphine alone, and the combination with 5 mg of amphetamine was 1.5 times as potent as morphine alone. In simple performance tests, and in measures of side effects, dextroamphetamine generally offsets undesirable morphine side effects of sedation and loss of alertness while increased analgesia. The effects on blood pressure, pulse, and respiratory rate were minimal. In this study a true synergism between these two compounds was proved for the first time in the human being. This same finding previously had been demonstrated in animal studies (Nickerson and Goodman 1947).

A study using a tourniquet pain technique has recently established the effectiveness of an orally administered combination of an opiate and an amphetamine. With the use of a double-blind technique, the experimenters compared placebo, anileridine at 25 mg, amphetamine at 10 mg, and anileridine at 25 mg plus amphetamine at 10 mg. Anileridine was used because it has a better absorbability than most opiates. Data confirmed that the time to unbearable pain was lengthened by the combination of the opiate plus the amphetamine compared with either the opiate alone or amphetamine alone. All drugs were significantly more effective than a placebo.

The results of all of these studies demonstrate that one can combine an amphetamine with an opiate, in either oral or injectable form, to produce a patient essentially free of pain with little sedation and few or no effects on vital signs, who is fully mentally capable, in a state of euphoria. Further, that even episodic doses of the drug mixture overcome the symptoms of depression. The utility of such a drug combination in the terminally ill is obvious. Indeed, the mixture of orally administered cocaine and heroin used at St. Christopher's Hospice (London) is an example of such use based on the same principles of pharmacology that underlie the studies of the amphetamines and opiates. Further, Houde of Sloan-Kettering Institute has used injectable forms of morphine and amphetamine mixtures with some of the terminally ill patients under his care.

The problem of the terminally ill patient in pain has always presented a dilemma. On one hand, we wish to provide adequate analgesia. On the other, we do not wish to hasten death by causing a depression of vital functions. Further, one would wish active, awake patients who are not depressed, who can communicate with their friends and family so that the act of dying will be minimally distressful and maximally dignified. The particular combination of drugs discussed in this paper would seeem to be of great benefit to this type of person. With an abundance of basic pharmacological and clinical data available to us on the proven utility of these combinations, it would appear to me that their general use should be quickly accepted.

References

Abel, S. and S. C. Harris. 1947. "Morphine-Benzedrine Analgesia in Obstetrics." Abstract of paper presented at proceedings of the American Physiological Society, p. 67.

Abel, S. B. Zelda, A. Ball, and S. C. Harris, 1951. "The Advantages to the Mother and Infant of Amphetamine in Obstetrical Analgesia." *American Journal of Obstetrics and Gynecology* 62:15.

Deneau, G. 1970. "Study of the Comparative Abuse Potentials of Dextroamphetamine, Morphine, and a Mixture of Dextroamphetamine plus Morphine." *Report to U.S. Army,* Contract No. DAAG 17-70-C-1152, Southern Research Institute, Birmingham, Alabama.

Evans, W. O. 1962. "The Synergism of Autonomic Drugs on Opiate or Opioid-Induced Analgesia: A Discussion of Its Potential Utility." *Military Medicine* 127:1000.

———. 1967. "The Effect of Stimulant Drugs on Opiate-Induced Analgesia." *Archives of Biological and Medical Experimentation* 4:144.

Evans, W. O., and R. P. Smith, 1964. "Some Effects of Morphine and Amphetamine on Intellectual Functioning and Mood." *Psychopharmacology* (Berlin) 6:49.

Forrest, W. H., J. W. Bellville, E. F. Beer, and B. W. Brown, 1970. "Interaction of Morphine and Dextroamphetamine for the Treatment of Postoperative Pain in Man." *Pharmacology* 12:210.

Forrest, W. H., B. W. Byron, C. R. Brown, R. Defalque, M. Gold, H. E. Gordon, K. E. James, J. Katz, D. L. Mahler, F. Schroff, and G. Teutsch, 1977. "Dextroamphetamine with Morphine for the Treatment of Postoperative Pain." *New England Journal of Medicine* 296:712.

Ivy, A. C., F. R. Goetzl, and D. Y. Burrill. 1944. "Morphine-Dextroamphetamine Analgesia." *War Medicine* 6:67.

Jasinski, D. R. and J. G. Nutt. 1972. "Progress Report on the Assessment Program of the NIMH Addiction Research Center." Committee on Problems of Drug Dependence, NAC, p. 442.

Lehmann, H. E., J. V. Ananth, K. L. Geagea, and T. A. Ban. 1971. "Treatment of Depression with Dexedrine and Demerol." *Current Therapeutic Research* 13:42.

Nickerson, M. 1950. "Analgesic Effects of Nitrous Oxide and Meperidine Alone and Combined with Amphetamine." *Western Social and Clinical Research,* April, p. 541.

Nickerson, M. and L. S. Goodman. 1947. "Synergistic Isonipecaine-Amphetamine Analgesia." *Federation Proceedings* 6:360.

Takagi, H., T. Takashima, and K. Kimura. 1964. "Antagonism of the Analgesic Effect of Morphine in Mice by Tetrabenazine and Reserpine." *Archives of Internal Pharmacodynamics* 149:484.

15.
PHARMACOKINETIC ASPECTS OF ANALGESIA DURING PALLIATIVE CARE

M. Keeri-Szanto

This paper focuses on the pharmacokinetic aspects of pain relief in problem patients. I define the objective of pain relief as alert analgesia; it is immaterial how much drug is required to achieve this. The problem patient can then be defined as one in whom it proves impossible to provide alert analgesia for the full length of a conventional dosing cycle, no matter what drug and what dosing strategy are employed. Such patients may then become candidates for more complex techniques of providing alert analgesia. It is my message that before these techniques (nerve blocks, tractotomies, hypnosis, transcendental meditation, LSD, etc.) are explored, one ought to investigate what demand analgesia has to offer these patients.

In the course of demand analgesia small narcotic increments are administered intravenously whenever the patient triggers the apparatus. It has certain disadvantages:

1. An intravenous line must be in place.
2. The apparatus is not portable by the patient in its present form and costs about $2,000 per unit.
3. Potentially lethal amounts of narcotics are attached to the patient at certain times, making it essential that the equipment function in a fail-safe fashion.

The advantages of such an approach are also considerable:

1. The patient modulates directly the number of drug increments received per unit time.

2. Delays between requests for medication and the appearance of the drug in the bloodstream are eliminated.

3. The use of small increments administered as frequently as 10 minutes apart, if necessary, eliminates the wide fluctuation of drug levels at the target site.

4. The procedure reduces anticipatory pain and the feeling of dependency and thus provides important psychological benefits for the patient.

5. The therapist can gain a much clearer understanding of the precipitating causes and the intensity of pain in a particular individual by studying the rate of self-administration than from the conventional requests for medication.

Equipment described by the author earlier (1971) has been in continuous use for many years and has shown no instance of technical malfunction. Although most of my experience was obtained in postoperative subjects (Keeri-Szanto and Herman 1972), I have also reported on the use of demand analgesia in the chronically or terminally ill (Keeri-Szanto 1976). My findings suggest that apparent habituation to narcotic action is often metabolic rather than pharmacological; i.e., the drug is metabolized more rapidly by such an individual while the sensitivity of the receptor site remains essentially unchanged. Such patients may be expected to show a high incidence of anticipatory pain, and ever smaller segments of the dosing cycle remain available for feeding, turning, contact with one's surroundings and relatives, and so forth. The institution of demand analgesia reaches the root of all these problems, and it should come as no surprise that it improves not just the quality but also the length of survival.

This procedure need not be reserved for the final weeks of life. With a little ingenuity, permanent intravenous sites can be created, and portable constant-infusion pumps that need to be recharged only once a week are currently available. Following initial titration, patients can be discharged from hospital with such a device in place when intractable pain was the only problem requiring hospitalization.

The problem of addiction is irrelevant in the terminal care of patients. Nevertheless, we found it comforting that the average patient, faced with the trade-off between obtunding the last vestige of pain or preserving alertness, unfailingly opts for alertness.

It is appreciated that intensity is not the only dimension of any type of pain, least of all during the terminal care of patients. Nevertheless, the other dimensions of pain cannot be successfully approached unless its intensity is under control; the reduction of pain intensity goes a long way toward controlling anticipatory pain, feelings of dependency, and so forth. This is particularly true if the patient can be made a participant in the process of pain control.

In summary, the decision of providing analgesia through drugs is based on the simplicity and economy of this technique. Its goal is to provide alert analgesia that promotes rather than hinders the physiological and psychological processes the patient must pass through on the road to a "good death." Pharmacological routes to alert analgesia should not be considered failures until all the options that arise from the pharmacokinetic peculiarities of a given drug in an individual patient are explored. Intravenous demand analgesia is one of these options.

References

Keeri-Szanto, M. 1971. "Apparatus for Demand Analgesia." *Canadian Anaesthesiology Society Journal* 18:581–82.

Keeri-Szanto, M. 1976. "Demand Analgesia for the Relief of Pain Problems in Terminal Illness." *Anesthesiology Review* 3:19–21.

Keeri-Szanto, M. and S. Herman. 1972. "Postoperative Demand Analgesia." *Surgery, Gynecology, and Obstetrics* 134:647–51.

16.
RELIEF FOR THE DYING AND THE BEREAVED: THE ROLE OF PSYCHOPHARMACOLOGIC AGENTS AND ANALGESICS

CHING-PIAO CHIEN, BALU KALAYAM,
AND REUBEN J. SILVER

Rationale of the Study

Although dying and grief are neglected entities, they are also the most dramatic stresses encountered by individuals in their lifetimes. If the pain and suffering of dying and grief should become intolerable or incapacitating, psychiatric intervention, including pharmacotherapy, should be considered, just as they would be for any emotional disorder. However, the ambivalence toward psychotropic drugs (Balter et al. 1974; Muller 1972) among certain populations may arouse psychological conflicts when psychopharmacologic agents and analgesics for the dying and the bereaved are prescribed.

The current national concern over drug abuse, particularly on overdependence on the mind-changing and analgesic agents, has generated fears concerning the weakening of the human mind and character (Balter et al. 1974; Muller 1972, Lennard et al. 1970). On the other hand, permission for physicians to use marijuana and other controlled substances in treating the terminally ill patient has been proposed at both national and state levels (*The New York Times* 1977; *New York State Medical Society*

1978). Given such a social background, we approached various professionals who deal with the dying and the bereaved, to determine their attitudes toward the use of psychopharmacologic and analgesic agents with this specific patient population.

Method

Subjects

Four groups in the capital district area of New York State were surveyed. Group 1 consisted of all physicians who were affiliated with local nursing homes. These are referred to as nursing home physicians (NHMD.) Group 2 consisted of all psychiatrists (PSYCH) affiliated with the Albany Medical College or who were listed under the heading "Psychiatrist" in the Albany telephone book. Group 3 were the paramedical mental health workers (MHW), composed of psychologists, social workers, nurses, and mental health aides who were employed by the Capital District Psychiatric Center and/or the Albany Medical Center. Group 4, the clergy, were 80 names selected at random from a list of 200 names in the *"Tri-City Area Council of Churches."*

The number of subjects surveyed and the number responding in each group is shown in table 16.1.

The response rate varied from a low of 47 percent for the nursing home physicians to a high of 87 percent for psychiatrists. Since all subjects were responding anonymously, breakdown by sex, age, or other parameter is possible.

Procedure

The questionnaire used to survey attitudes is presented in table 16.2. It consisted of 10 items, scored on a seven-point

Table 16.1. Number of Subjects Surveyed and the Number Responding

Group	Number Surveyed	Number Responding	Percentage Responding
NHMD.	70	33	47%
PSYCH	60	52	87%
MHW	150	81	54%
CLERGY	80	45	56%
Total	360	211	58%

rating scale, which ranged from 1, strongly agree, to 7, strongly disagree. The items are shown in table 16.2.

This questionnaire and a covering letter were sent to the subjects in the four groups. Since anonymity of the person answering the survey was maintained, it is not possible to do any follow-up requests to increase the percentage responding. Group membership of the subject was revealed by colorcoding the answer sheets.

Table 16.2. Questionnaire

Q 1. *Analgesic* agents should be administered to the *dying patients* who are in pain.
Q 2. *Addiction* or a constant state of lethargy caused by analgesics and/or narcotics should not be considered *contraindications* for administering these drugs to *dying patients*.
Q 3. *Antianxiety* agents should be administered to the *dying patient* for *anxiety symptoms*.
Q 4. *Antidepressants* should be administered to the *dying patient* for *depressive symptoms*.
Q 5. *Antipsychotics* should be administered to the *dving patient* for *psychotic breakdown*.
Q 6. The *grief* of the bereaved should be permitted to run its *natural course* rather than dealt with by drug intervention.
Q 7. The *emotional disturbance* of the *bereaved* should be treated with *antianxiety agents* for anxiety symptoms.
Q 8. The *emotional disturbance* of the *bereaved* should be treated with *antidepressants* for depressive symptoms.
Q 9. The *emotional disturbance* of the *bereaved* should be treated with *antipsychotics* for psychotic symptoms.
Q 10. Philosophically, when *death is inevitable*, the *natural course* should be preferred instead of maintaining the life of the patient through rigorous interventions.

(Response key: 1 = strongly agree, 2 = moderately agree, 3 = mildly agree, 4 = neither agree nor disagree, 5 = mildly disagree, 6 = moderately disagree, 7 = strongly disagree).

Results

Means and standard deviations for the four groups on each of the 10 items are shown in table 16.3. It can be seen that all groups were positive in their attitudes toward the use of drugs with the dying patient. Although the clergy were more negative toward medication, they too tended to the positive end of the scale on questions concerning the treatment of the dying patient.

The attitudes toward the use of specific psychopharmacologic agents for the bereaved are of particular interest. When the question dealt with anxiety, depression, and psychosis, the mean ratings for all groups approached the middle of the scale (neither agree nor disagree) except for the favorable attitude of psychiatrists toward using an antipsychotic drug in cases of psychotic breakdown. All groups exhibited significant variations over using drugs to treat the bereaved.

Differences among group responses to the questionnaire were analyzed by one way analysis of variance (table 16.4), which revealed significant F-tests on all but two of the items, viz., the use of antidepressants for the bereaved who were depressed and the philosophical issue regarding the preference of natural course for death without vigorous intervention.

The results of Newman-Keuls Tests done on all items in which the groups had significant F-tests are given in table 16.5.

Table 16.3. Means and Standard Deviations of the Four Groups for the Ten Questionnaire Items

Group	NHMD		PSYCH		MHW		CLERGY	
Item	M.	S.D.	M.	S.D.	M.	S.D.	M.	S.D.
Pain in dying	1.03	0.17	1.33	1.2	1.23	0.65	1.73	0.94
Addiction	1.52	0.94	1.65	1.31	2.26	1.76	3.49	2.16
Anxiety in dying	1.88	1.18	1.78	1.45	2.15	1.58	3.33	2.06
Depression in dying	1.93	1.18	2.13	1.72	2.63	1.98	3.25	2.01
Psychosis in dying	2.15	1.38	1.53	1.29	1.82	1.30	2.36	1.60
Grief in bereaved	3.32	2.07	3.06	1.81	2.83	1.76	1.93	1.26
Anxiety in bereaved	2.90	1.72	3.12	1.76	3.32	1.80	4.45	1.77
Depression in bereaved	3.03	1.80	3.34	2.19	3.82	1.95	4.11	1.63
Psychosis in bereaved	2.50	1.84	1.92	1.52	2.30	1.76	3.18	1.76
Natural death	1.39	0.89	1.88	1.36	1.81	1.32	1.35	1.09

Table 16.4. One-Way Analysis of Variance of Four Groups' Scores on Ten Questionnaire Items

Item	F Test	p
1. Pain in dying	5.00	<.002
2. Addiction	12.77	<.000
3. Anxiety in dying	8.85	<.000
4. Depression in dying	4.29	<.006
5. Psychosis in dying	3.20	<.024
6. Grief in bereaved	4.99	<.000
7. Anxiety in bereaved	6.42	<.000
8. Depression in bereaved	2.58	>.054
9. Psychosis in bereaved	4.45	<.005
10. Natural death	2.40	>.068

Inspection of that table reveals that there were no significant differences between the nursing home physicians and the psychiatrists on any of the items.

Mental health workers differed significantly from nursing home physicians and from psychiatrists on only one item, viz., usage of antidepressants for depressive symptoms in the dying patients.

The clergy differed significantly from the other groups on 8 of the 10 items. In general, the clergy tended to be less favorable toward drug intervention than the other three groups; how-

Table 16.5. Results of Student-Newman-Keuls Significance Tests for Ten Questionnaire Items

Item	Newman-Keuls Results
1. Pain in dying	D > A, B, C*
2. Addiction	D > A, B, C
3. Anxiety in dying	D > A, B, C
4. Depression in dying	D > C > B, A
5. Psychosis in dying	D > B
6. Grief in bereaved	D > A, B, C
7. Anxiety in bereaved	D > A, B, C
8. Depression in bereaved	No significant differences
9. Psychosis in bereaved	D > B, C
10. Natural death	No significant differences

*CODE
A: Nursing home physicians
B: Psychiatrists
C: Mental health workers
D: Clergy

Significant differences (.05 level) between group means are indicated by the symbol > or <.

ever, the clergy did not differ from the other three professional groups on two items, administering antidepressants for the bereaved and the philosophical preference of natural death.

It is interesting that in item 10—a philosophical question dealing with attitudes toward death—all groups concurred in the opinion that when death is inevitable, the natural course is to be preferred over maintaining the life of the patient through vigorous intervention.

Discussion

Although the clergy showed the least favorable attitude toward the use of drugs and even objected slightly to using antianxiety and antidepressant agents for the bereaved, their overall scores were mostly within the agreeable category in terms of usage of drugs, and they agreed strongly that analgesic agents should be administered to dying patients who are in pain. Therefore, differences among the four groups should be viewed as a quantitative rather than qualitative difference. What is needed, then, is information regarding the consumer's attitude—which was not measured in this phase of our study, for logistical reasons. In the next phase, attempts will be made to survey the attitude of the patient, dying and not dying, and of his family. We hope thus to achieve a better understanding of the variables that affect the consumer's attitude toward drug therapy.

Special clinical consideration should be given to the consumer during drug treatment, particularly in situations where attitude data are lacking. Despite the beneficial effects of psychopharmacologic and analgesic drugs, their side effects, which may distort bodily functions, may cause unnecessary alarm and panic to the already distressed dying or bereaved person. For example, dystonia may be misperceived as convulsions, akathisia as agony, postural hypotension as impending stroke drowsiness as losing consciousness; etc. Advance explanation, assurance, and rapid management of such side effects require special clinical consideration.

Since side effects vary from person to person, and since individual attitudes toward drugs and psychological reactions to side effects depend significantly on each individual's psychosocial and cultural-religious background, medication requires more careful, individual tailoring than is the case in regular clinical practice. Medication may generally be handled by the family physician, or by a nonpsychiatric specialist; yet when the patient manifests a strong emotional reaction to the pharmacological approach, it is advisable to consult with a psychiatrist with good knowledge of psychopharmacology, rather than to withdraw drug treatment abruptly. The psychiatrist may identify some hidden psychological issue that accounts for the patient's reaction to drug therapy, and thus potentiate a more rational therapeutic approach.

Summary

Despite the significant medical contribution of modern pharmacotherapy, there is national concern lest the wide usage of psychotropic drugs and narcotics will weaken the human mind in a "drug-culture" society. The psychological needs of the dying and the bereaved have been acknowledged only in recent years. What, then, is the optimal role of psychopharmacologic and analgesic agents in relieving the dying and the bereaved, as compared with their use in managing other emotional stresses? The current study is designed to explore the attitudes of four different professional groups who are often involved in dealing with these special cases.

A total of 211 professionals representing four groups (nursing home physicians, psychiatrists, paramedical mental health workers, and clergy) from the capital district area of New York State responded to a specially designed 10 item questionnaire exploring their attitude toward the use of antianxiety, antidepressant, antipsychotic, and analgesic agents for the corresponding symptoms in the dying and the bereaved.

The results revealed that although clergy consistently showed a "least favorable" attitude toward the use of drugs, all four groups were in agreement with using these agents in their overall scores. Thus, the difference among the four groups should be considered as quantitative rather than qualitative. Emphasis is placed on special clinical and individual considerations in dealing with the panic and fear caused by the occasional side effects of these drugs.

References

Balter, M. B., J. Levine, and D. I. Manheimer. 1974. "Cross-national Study of the Extent of Anti-anxiety/Sedative Drug Use." *New England Journal of Medicine* 290:769–74.
"Bills That Would Permit Physicians To Administer Heroin." 1978. *News of New York (Medical Society of the State of New York)* 33(7):3.
Lennard, H. L., L. J. Epstein, A. Bernstein, et al. 1970. "Hazards Implicit in Prescribing Psychoactive Drugs." *Science* 169:438–41.
Muller, C. 1972. "The Over-medicated Society—Forces in the Market Place for Medical Care." *Science* 176:488–92.
"Panel To Examine the Way U.S. Deals with Dying People." 1977. *The New York Times*, November 17.

17.
THE CANCER WARD

Irene B. Seeland

The increase in knowledge about treating cancer patients with chemotherapy and radiation therapy has enabled us to extend people's lives but has also produced considerable stress and complications within the therapeutic environment. There is a longer period of time for awareness that the illness will be progressive, that preparations for death should be made. There are socioeconomic problems for patients and their families because families are left with fairly critical economic stresses at the end of an extended progressive illness. Many times patients who have been the main provider in the family or the household caretaker become increasingly unable to work as debilitation sets in. The stresses on everybody involved in the cancer situation are extreme and add to the already existing trauma induced by the illness itself. As the symptoms and disabilities of disease increase throughout the period when life is being extended through the use of chemotherapy, many people—patients, families, and physicians—have difficulty in coping with one or another aspect of life as it is.

But what actually happens on a larger cancer treatment ward? The ward on which I have been the psychiatric consultant has been open for four years and has a very active treatment population. All the patients are on chemotherapy protocols and usually do not stay for long periods of time. Most are discharged after a brief stay but return for additional chemotherapy or for the treatment of complications, many of these stemming from the chemotherapy.

I would like to describe a study (not in the format of a protocol) that was performed concerning the kinds of medications being used and the effects of these on the status and pain of the life-threatened patient, families, and staff. Over a period of five weeks, on every other week, the patients on the ward and their pain medication, as well as any tranquilizers or antidepressants being prescribed, were reviewed. To a large degree, the patients on this ward are cared for by their private physicians, oncologists with expertise in dealing with cancer patients. All approach the treatment of their particular patients from the perspective of their own individual experiences, so that the result of therapy does not reflect an agreed-upon pain protocol. Yet very interesting findings came out of our brief study.

Thirty-three patients were reviewed. Seventeen were between the ages of 45 and 65, stricken at a very active time in their lives, most of them still working and many with adolescent children. Six were younger (under 30), and ten were over 65. Actually, all had anticipated many more years of life before the confrontation with an illness that would predictably shorten their life expectancy. Fourteen percent had solid tumors—of the lung, breast, colon, pancreas, and head and neck—many of these already metastatic to bone. There were a number of patients with lymphomas, Hodgkins disease, and acute and chronic leukemias. Those patients who actually complained about pain were in the minority, nine of the 33.

My review concentrated on the patients who felt in need of ongoing pain medication. Those medications requested and used most frequently were Tylenol and Dalmane, the former for pain and fever and the latter as a sleeping medication. Aspirin could not be used on the cancer ward, because every patient suffered from bone marrow depression caused by the chemotherapeutic agents, and aspirin acts to further decrease the bone marrow. Nearly half of the patients were using these medications as their primary mode of treatment, but only nine were in serious need of ongoing, round-the-clock medication.

Of the actual analgesics used, I was surprised to find that only three patients were on morphine or Demerol and that the other patients on pain medication were on Dilaudid, a morphine derivative that can be used orally, or codeine, or codeine and a combination of other medications. Both medical and nursing staffs felt that these medications were appropriate for this patient population because they could be administered orally. Round-the-clock injections would have caused both bleeding and excessive pain because of the patients' low platelet counts. Four to six injections a day for a patient who may have a hematoma at each injection site can be excruciating physically for the patient and most stressful for the nurse who has to administer them.

Seven patients had used Valium, but not on a regular basis. Most of these patients had the medication available, for it was often given before tests to reduce anxiety. (The experience of being summoned for a test and then waiting for an indefinite period in the testing area was extremely anxiety producing. If a patient did not know what the test entailed, a consent form had to be signed.) Other patients were on medications like chlorpromazine and trimethobenzamide which have tranquilizing effects but are usually utilized to avoid vomiting or hiccoughs—specific symptoms in many patients with uremia. Three patients were on no medication, for at their stage of the disease, no acute discomfort was in evidence.

I explored those medications used freely in other institutions but only on a limited basis on our ward. Brompton's Mixture, available and recommended highly by those who had worked in other hospices with patients in continuous need of medication, was an example of these. I found that the morphine sulfate in our Brompton's "cocktail" induced fairly severe gastric reactions in certain patients. Another problem involved in its use came from the fact that the prescription could be filled only from the hospital pharmacy, and the nurses felt hesitant about recommending it for patients who were to be discharged. The prescription was not renewable elsewhere, and the patients would have to wait for three or four hours in the pharmacy outpatient line to have a prescription filled. This was a matter of crucial importance for the discharged patient who might need any kind of medication repeatedly.

Another analgesic presenting somewhat similar problems was methadone, which can be prescribed in this country for medical reasons. It was found that patients had very strong feelings about methadone use because of its association with the treatment of heroin addiction. This particular problem is confirmed by the following illustration:

> A young black woman, a 30-year-old nurse, had advanced metastatic breast cancer, with disease spread to her arms and skin. She was being treated on an outpatient basis in the oncology clinic. A strong, competent person, she lived in a fairly poor area of Harlem. One day when she came to the clinic, she appeared to be very upset. Although it was a fairly cold day, perspiration was running down her face. I asked her, "Are you in pain?" And she started to cry. "Yes," she answered, "I am in extreme pain." When I asked her why she had not said something before, she replied, "I'm so afraid of becoming addicted. I don't want to become addicted." I explained that there are medications she would not have to worry about becoming addicted to as well as the fact that, from her social background, it was natural for her to have exaggerated fears about what any kind of analgesic might lead to. After we worked these facts through, she was able to accept pain medication and live in comfort until her death a short time later.

It is unfortunate that mixed messages about addiction come to both patients and physicians in times of duress. It must be accepted that it is all right to take morphine, Demerol, or other potentially addictive medication to relieve extreme pain.

It was surprising to note that none of our patients were on antidepressants although obviously some of them were struggling with difficult emotional issues. In staff discussions held regularly, it became evident that our approach to patients—relating to them so that we could establish adequate support systems within the hospital, outside of the hospital, and with their families—relieved their anxieties about reality issues far more effectively than prescribing antidepressants.

The nursing staff were very sensitive to and acutely aware of the needs of the patients. Our system assigned a specific nurse to a specific patient. The nurse then knew the patient very well and many times also knew the family. Within such a setting, the nurse is able to acquire a fairly comprehensive understanding of the psychosocial situation affecting patients and families. Over a period of time and recurrent hospitalizations, a staff member can follow the history of the family. The nurse often intervened as a mental health worker, and crisis intervention and supportive work were possible, and these reduced the need for psychotropic medication. It is a fact that human contact provides better relief for anxiety than drugs do.

It is, however, apparent that the nurse cannot do everything, that the whole patient care concept in most hospitals needs revising, and that the education of medical staff should stress the role of the physician and others as healers, comforters, and givers of support. With increased interest in ethical issues by caregivers, the care given to the terminal patient—the patient on the cancer ward—takes on a different dimension. More than emotional anxiety will be tempered. There is little doubt that physical suffering also responds dramatically to therapeutic measures other than those agents prescribed for the relief of pain.

18.
PHARMACOLOGIC AGENTS: BARRIERS OR TOOLS?

Samuel C. Klagsbrun

We are so successful in pain control that we must think about the complications of our success. Pharmacologic agents are tools that now allow us to go back to the original position many of us were in when we started treating dying patients or patients with pain. We have a built-in barrier that allows us to return to a kind of distance between ourselves and our patients. We rationalize the distance by thinking that we are doing good.

The purpose of medication relates *to* relieving pain. We want our patients to be relatively free of crippling depressions and anxiety. These goals are realistic and sensible.

But here is an example of the *irony* of the effective use of medication. Barry is now 16 years old. Approximately 10 years ago, the diagnosis of leukemia was made. His parents decided, under the advice of their physician, not to tell Barry about the nature of his illness. They used the usual euphemisms—a bad cold that affects joints—a fancy name like lymphadenitis to give a sense of respectability. About a year after diagnosis, Barry overheard his mother discussing leukemia on the phone. Barry went to his parents' study and pulled out a volume of the *World Book*. His mother found him looking at the L's in the encyclopedia and recognized that it was time to have a discussion with Barry. An approximation of the truth was given to him.

Barry was treated for 10 years on various protocols. Six months ago, as an adolescent, he was pronounced "cured" because he was taken off all protocols and was symptom free and feeling fine. Barry was no longer treated for cancer. During the 10-year period he received medications for psychological reasons, pain reasons (when necessary), and certainly for the treatment of leukemia.

About a month ago, Barry attempted suicide. The reason for the attempt had to do with the impact of cancer on his life. He was a developing young man who felt different and alienated from other kids. Though he was now pronounced "cured," he was left feeling defenseless from spending so much time away from others because of hospitalizations and restrictions on activities. For Barry, reentry into adolescent society was an overwhelmingly frightening task. He felt that he was not up to it.

Barry was in constant communication in the sense that his family was open. He had psychiatric treatment to help him overcome gaps between the normal adolescent's development and the life he was leading. Barry had as much support as one could realistically offer any single human being going through this problem. Yet Barry wanted to die.

When we pieced things together, it became clear that one inadequate area of Barry's experience with cancer was the primary physician's care. For ten years, the importance of Barry's oncologist to him was so great that discharge literally meant being abandoned by that doctor. The doctor had been quite sensitive and effective, and in a way that was his problem. He was aware of the importance of what he said to Barry. For 10 years he had been careful about the way he treated Barry. He used medications carefully and explained the impact of each one. Barry was fully prepared during the treatment—except for the doctor's leaving him.

We must recognize that we, the givers of chemotherapeutic, pharmacologic, or psychopharmalogic agents, are the real agents in the relationships with people who are dying. The doctor in Barry's case considered himself important to Barry because he was giving the proper drugs. But what Barry saw was a human being who cared about him and who (secondarily) occasionally bothered him with nauseating medications. So, in thinking about psychopharmacologic agents for the treatment of cancer, we have to pay careful attention that the agents do not work alone.

Communications are enhanced when one uses medications properly. In a peculiar way, as a psychiatrist, I am now focusing on a dimension I am most comfortable with—people-to-people contact. Psychopharmacologic agents are helping agents, entities for improved communications.

The purpose of using drugs is to help people remain alive, in touch with families, friends, and feelings. Once such a person feels sadness, frustration, and pain, one has possibly created a source of aggravation. If really alive, the person will obviously be angry at the situation. Once one starts giving drugs to help someone remain alive, one must offer a support system aiding families and friends to tolerate all that the patient says and demands. Otherwise, in the area of medication, one will face what happens with some juvenile diabetics and other difficult patients—acting out, forgetting medications, overdosing medications (all relating to the unconscious wish of many families and patients to be rid of being alive).

Another example is Eric, a young man with glioblastoma. During the course of psychotherapy, Eric developed double vision and headaches. After strongly urging him repeatedly to see a physician, I simply took him next door to the neurologist and said, "You're seeing this doctor right now." Unfortunately the need for that step became evident. Eric is dying right now.

The doctor to whom I took Eric is extremely competent. However, he is unable to communicate effectively with Eric. Eric continues to see me, and I have become a translator for the neurologist and for the neurosurgeon.

Eric is on medications that include cortisone. Every time Eric calls his neurologist, the neurologist increases medications appropriately. Then Eric calls me and asks for my explanation of the effects of the increasing doses. I give him the information and then he feels better.

A few weeks ago I asked Eric why he doesn't ask his doctor these questions. Eric said he thinks that the doctor is irritated with him because he is not a good patient. ("I'm dying and the doctor doesn't like that.") Eric said that whenever he speaks to

Pharmacologic Agents: Barriers or Tools?

his doctor about that kind of subject (dying), the doctor says, "No—you do not have a malignancy. You have a kind of tumor that can grow back again and we may have to continue your treatment. But you do not have cancer."

Then Eric came back to me and asked, "What do I have?" and I answered, "You have cancer." Eric responded, "I know that. Why isn't the doctor able to talk about it?" We get into this kind of a hassle where medications are the focus of communication between patient and doctor.

Eric's case may be an extreme example. Although Eric will continue to have increasing loss of trust in his doctor, he is able to do something sophisticated—separate the person of that doctor from his technical competence. And he has done what many patients do.

That a patient accepts pharmacologic agents from the physician does not mean that there is a good situation, relationship, or series of contacts. What we may have is acceptance of someone's technical aspect but rejection of the rest. This is a sad commentary on the nature of some cancer treatment.

I have been involved with an experimental cancer patient group. It is group therapy, and the "ticket of admission" is having cancer. Eight women were together for a year and a half.

The reason for the group was one woman—a character actress with metastasized breast cancer. She felt that it simply was not enough to be alive and to be receiving chemotherapy. She wanted something more effective, and she knew of my interest.

The group talked about life and focused on what it is like to face the routine problems of living when one has cancer, when one is treated for it, and when one spends two days vomiting every two weeks. We talked about what one does if one is a character actress on Broadway whose hair is falling out. How does one feel about wearing a wig in the summer if one has rivers of sweat streaming out from underneath one's wig in a nonairconditioned place?

Patients in the group exchanged vital information about chemotherapy and the latest pain control medications. I learned more there than I had from professional circles about nutritional experimentation and about oddball things. As a strong opponent of laetrile I was under periodic attack by the group.

Pharmacologic agents were extensively discussed and anger was expressed when members of the group believed that their physicians held back (on information, complications, amounts used, doses required). They wanted to know everything there was to know about management of cancer.

The women are now back into life, having sex, getting married (in that order), taking driving lessons, traveling around the world, pushing for careers, running for office. They are an incredibly vital group.

Something else is happening that I do not understand. They are all getting better, even though these people have extensive metastatic disease. The founding member of the group, the actress, has gone from an inoperable carcinoma to—literally—no palpable lumps. Her well-known oncologist does not understand why his treatment has been so successful. I do not understand either.

Perhaps pharmacologic agents have been used in these instances as means for bringing patients back into living, into the normal complications and aggravations of life. The agents have not been used as barriers that allow us to remain hidden behind our white coats.

19.
PSYCHOLOGICAL RESPONSES IN THE DYING PATIENT: A ROLE FOR BEHAVIORALLY ACTIVE PEPTIDE HORMONES?

Daniel Carr

Published accounts of the experiences of persons resuscitated after cardiorespiratory arrest have called attention to striking similarities between the experiences of many different individuals (Moody 1975, Osis and Haroldsson 1977). Increasing attention has focused on such accounts as providing concrete evidence of the existence of life after life (Stevenson and Greyson 1979). Because of the potentially profound implications of such accounts, it is important to assess them critically and in particular to ask whether plausible alternative explanations may be offered for the genesis of such psychological responses. In this brief paper I begin by viewing such responses as neurologic events, then consider which brain areas may underlie such events, and finally offer a novel explanation for the selective activation of these areas in near-death.

Passivity and analgesia have long been recognized as common among the terminally ill. Surveys have, however, identified an additional and distinct core group of complex psychological responses recollected by survivors of near-death experiences and also reported by lucid individuals in the preterminal state. These responses include euphoria, involuntary recall of memories, a sense of dissociation from one's body, and auditory, visual, or olfactory hallucinations (Moody 1975, Osis and Haraldsson 1977, Stevenson and Greyson 1979). If an otherwise healthy individual were to tell a physician that these mental changes occurred at unpredictable intervals, the physician would probably describe them as a "limbic lobe syndrome" and undertake medical tests to rule out a tumor or epileptic disorder involving these brain areas, which regulate mood and memory. Brain structures comprising the limbic system include the hypothalamus, hippocampus, septum, amygdala, portions of the cerebral cortex, and the reticular formation of the midbrain (Martin et al. 1977). The temporal lobe of the cerebral cortex is a major source of input to the hippocampus, and patients who suffer from paroxysms of neuronal discharge within the temporal lobe may report psychological aberrations including quasi-religious auras, feelings of deja-vu or jamais-vu, unprovoked feelings of rage or bliss, or frank hallucinations (Merritt 1973). Animals in which hippocampal seizures have been induced are described as appearing "catatonic" with waxy flexibility and immobility during periods of intense hippocampal activity (Henriksen et al. 1978). Dysfunction of other brain areas outside the limbic system would be expected to produce other characteristic signs: paralysis or selective anesthesia if the spinal cord were involved; slurring of speech, frank convulsions, blindness or partial paralysis with damage to motor or visual cortex; clumsiness or slurring of speech with cerebellar damage; impairment of consciousness with brain stem damage; and disorders of movement with disrupted basal ganglia function (Merritt 1973). Yet none of the latter symptom complexes seem to occur with regularity in the terminal state. Thus clinical correlations lend credence to the occurrence of a distinctive form of limbic lobe syndrome in many instances of near-death.

The understanding of limbic lobe physiology has been revolutionized in recent years by discoveries of peptide hormones within the brain. By now their story has been widely told: many reports have described how vasopressin plays a role in learning and memory and how fragments of the common precursor for ACTH and beta-endorphin modulate attention and play a crucial role in the reward pathways of the brain (Krieger and Hughes 1980). Less emphasis has been placed on the unique ability of beta-endorphin to provoke selective excitation of limbic lobe neurons, but ample experimental data confirm this striking property, at least in animal models (Gahwiler and Herring 1981, Lewis et al. 1981). As noted, animals undergoing hippocampal seizures resulting from the direct administration of opioid peptides within the brain do not show overt signs of convulsive activity; rather, they appear "catatonic" (Henriksen et al. 1978). Any relevance of animal studies to clinical phenomena is of course highly speculative; more relevant perhaps is a report of the infusion into cerebrospinal fluid of beta-endorphin in a group of patients suffering from severe pain due to cancer (Oyama et al. 1980). These patients reported not only analgesia but also, frequently, elevations of mood, yet had a minimal degree of other physical signs—such as pupillary constriction or respiratory depression—normally expected with opiate therapy. Postmortem studies in animals and human beings have shown high concentrations of opioid peptides within the limbic lobe (Rossier et al. 1977), as well as dense clusterings of the receptors for these hormones in the same area (Kuhar et al. 1973). Thus data now available are fragmentary and, while consistent with our hypothesis that behaviorally active peptides trigger a characteristic limbic lobe syndrome in terminal illness, by no means confirm it.

A separate line of evidence, derived from studies on stress, points strongly toward marked changes in brain metabolism of behaviorally active peptides, particularly beta-endorphin and related compounds, during potentially fatal illnesses. No more potent stimuli exist for the release of beta-endorphin and related compounds than a sudden decline in blood pressure (Gann et al. 1978), whether due to hemorrhage, sepsis, heart failure, or obstructed blood flow. This statement must be qualified by the recognition that measurements of blood levels of such hormones reflect release from the pituitary gland, which hangs from the brain, rather than from the brain itself. Studies to correlate declines in brain content of these peptides with their pituitary depletion have been few but do in fact suggest a fairly good correlation (Wardlaw and Frantz 1980). Other studies have examined the precise time course of the release of behaviorally active peptides from pituitary and brain in relation to stimuli such as hypotension or fever (Hamilton et al. 1981). Concomitantly, investigators have demonstrated increased survival in animals treated with narcotic antagonists before hemorrhage (Faden and Holaday 1979) or sepsis (Holaday and Faden 1978), and clinical practitioners are in the process of extending these findings to the medical treatment of shock (Dirksen et al. 1980). A further indirect piece of evidence for hypersecretion of ACTH and cosynthesized peptides (which include beta-endorphin) at the time of death is to be found in older findings of elevations of adrenal steroids shortly before death due to a variety of causes (Perkoff et al. 1954); adrenal steroid production is a marker of ACTH activity.

To summarize, one may interpret clinically the symptom complex described in many near-death experiences as reflecting altered limbic lobe function; it is likely that peptide hormones within the brain mediate this alteration of limbic lobe function; and it is probable that the physical circumstances of potentially fatal illness are sufficient stimuli for calling these compounds into action. Are there any precedents for such a model?

Emerging evidence points to the participation of multiple peptide hormones, including beta-endorphin, in the control of some crucial adjustments that occur at the time of birth, such as the initiation of spontaneous breathing (Wardlaw et al. 1979, Hazinski et al 1981). Just as respiratory reflexes are evoked whether birth occurs by spontaneous delivery or Caesarean section, so one may view the release of behaviorally active hormones as a feature in general of the transition from life to death regardless of the precise route taken (Carr 1983).

Every clinician has been impressed by instances where patients foresaw the day or time of their death and by the feelings reported by patients who have survived a brush with death. Frequently their feelings are of such vividness as to induce permanent, major changes in their perceptions and beliefs (Moody 1975, Osis and Haraldsson 1977, Stevenson and Greyson 1979). To unravel the pathophysiology of these psychological responses would not be easy but would be worthwhile. To my knowledge, the idea that reflexes may be evoked in the process of dying—just as other reflexes are evoked in the process of being born—is a novel one. However, the elucidation of perinatal reflexes has led to improved medical therapies, certainly has saved many lives, and is eminently worthy of pursuit. Perhaps the elucidation of previously unstudied reflexes of the moribund state may also result in unsuspected means of enhancing life.

Acknowledgments.

Support for the preparation of this manuscript was provided in part by NIH grant AM 07028–06. Stimulating discussions with Dr. Stephen Gullo of The Foundation of Thanatology catalyzed the ideas expressed here.

References

Carr, D. 1983. "Pathophysiology of Stress-Induced Limbic Lobe Dysfunction: A Hypothesis for NDEs." *Anabiosis—The Journal for Near-Death Studies* 3:75–89.
Dirksen, R. M., H. Otten, G. J. Wood, C. J. Verbaan, M. M. P. Haalebos, P. V. Verdouw, and G. M. M. Nijhhuis. 1980. "Naloxone in Shock." *Lancet* 2:1360–61.
Faden, A. I. and J. W. Holaday. 1979. "Opiate Antagonists: A Role in the Treatment of Hypovolemic Shock." *Science* 205:317–18.
Gahwiler, B. H. and P. C. Herring. 1981. "Effects of Opioid Peptides on Synaptic Potentials in Explants of Rat Hippocampus." *Regulatory Peptides* 1:317–26.
Gann, D. S., D. G. Ward, and D. R. Carlson. 1978. "Neural Control of ACTH: A Homeostatic Reflex." *Recent Progress in Hormone Research* 34:357–400.
Hamilton, A., D. Carr, M. Arnold, S. Lantos, M. Rosenblatt, J. T. Potts, Jr., and R. M. Bergland. 1981. *Clinical Research* 29:505A.
Hazinski, T. A., M. M. Grunstein, M. A. Schlueter, and W. H. Tooley. 1981. "Effect of Naloxone on Ventilation in Newborn Rabbits." *Journal of Applied Physiology* 50:713–17.
Henriksen, S., F. Bloom, F. McCoy, N. Ling, and R. Guillemin. 1978. "Beta-endorphin Produces Non-Convulsive Limbic Seizures." *Proceedings of the National Academy of Science of the United States* 75:5221–25.

Holaday, J. W. and A. I. Faden. 1978. "Naloxone Reversal of Endotoxin Hypotension Suggests Role of Endorphins in Shock." *Nature* 275:450–51.

Krieger, D. T. and J. C. Hughes, eds. 1980. *Neuroendocrinology*. New York: HP Publishing Co.

Kuhar, M. J., C. B. Pert, and S. H. Snyder. 1973. "Regional Distribution of Opiate Receptor Binding in Monkey and Human Brain." *Nature* 245:447–50.

Lewis, J. W., S. Caldecott-Hazard, J. T. Cannon, and J. C. Liebeskind. 1981. "Possible Role of Opioid Peptides in Pain Inhibition and Seizures." In J. B. Martin, S. Reichlin, and K. Bick., eds., *Neurosecretion and Brain Peptides*, New York: Raven.

Martin, J. B., S. Reuchlin, and G. M. Brown. 1977. *Clinical Neuroendocrinology*. Philadelphia: Davis.

Merritt, H. H. 1973. *A Textbook of Neurology* (fifth edition). Philadelphia: Lea and Febiger.

Moody, R. A. 1975. *Life After Life*. New York: Bantam.

Osis, K. and E. Haraldsson. 1977. *At the Hour of Death*. New York: Avon.

Oyama, T., T. Jin, R. Yama, N. Ling, and R. Guillemin. 1980. "Profound Analgesic Effects of Beta-Endorphin in Man." *Lancet* 1:122–24.

Perkoff, G. T., A. A. Sandberg, D. H. Nelson, and F. H. Tyler. 1954. "Clinical Usefulness of Determination of Circulating 17-hydroxycorticosteroid Levels." *Journal of the American Medical Association* 93:1–8.

Rossier, J., T. M. Vargo, S. Minick. N. Ling, F. E. Bloom, and R. Guillemin. 1977. "Regional Dissociation of Beta-endorphin and Enkephalin Contents in Rat Brain and Pituitary." *Proceedings of the National Academy of Science of USA* 74:5162–65.

Stevenson, I. and B. Greyson. 1979. "Near-Death Experiences: Relevance to the Question of Survival After Death." *Journal of the American Medical Association* 242:265–67.

Wardlaw, S. L. and A. G. Frantz. 1980. "Effect of Swimming Stress on Brain Beta-endorphin and ACTH." *Clinical Research* 28:482A.

Wardlaw, S. L., R. I. Stark, L. Baxi, and A. G. Frantz. 1979. "Plasma Beta-endorphin and Beta-lipotropin in the Human Fetus at Delivery: Correlation with Arterial pH and pO_2." *Journal of Clinical Endocrinology and Metabolism* 49:888–91.

III.
RELIEVING THE GRIEF AND ANXIETY OF BEREAVEMENT

20.
ACUTE GRIEF: A PHYSICIAN'S VIEWPOINT

Robert G. Twycross

Acute grief is characterized by recurrent episodes of severe anxiety and psychological pain during which the dead person is strongly missed and the survivor sobs or cries aloud for him or her. These "pangs of grief" begin within a few hours or days of bereavement and usually reach a peak of severity within five to fourteen days. Initially, they occur frequently and spontaneously. Parkes (1972) writes:

> Feelings of pain, a dry mouth and other indications of automatic activity are particularly pronounced during pangs of grief. Add to these features deep sighing respiration, restless but aimless hyperactivity, difficulty in concentrating on anything but thoughts of loss, ruminations around the events leading up to the loss as well as loss of interest in any of the people or things that normally give pleasure or claim attention, and one begins to get a picture of this distressing phase of grief.

The Use of Psychopharmacologic Agents

In view of this catalog of symptoms, it is not surprising that many people consult their doctor in the months after bereavement. Indeed, in the United Kingdom, where it is common for all members of a family to be cared for by a single practitioner within the National Health Service, a growing number of doctors regard visiting the newly bereaved as part of their routine.

In this situation what help should the doctor offer? In particular, to what extent should the use of psychopharmacologic agents be encouraged? Benjamin Rush, famous American physician and signatory of the Declaration of Independence, advised the prescription of "liberal doses of opium." Today, he would no doubt recommend equally liberal doses of barbiturates or benzodiazepine tranquilizers. Kübler-Ross (1973) has denounced this type of approach, suggesting instead that we should establish a "screaming room" where the unexpectedly bereaved could sit and cry and scream in the presence of an understanding listening nurse or minister. She believes that we could take care of these people with much less medication and thus enable them to face the painful reality fully conscious and without feelings of shame or embarrassment. If, despite this sort of approach, sedation still appears necessary, it should be given, but in a dose that does not leave the bereaved person feeling drugged or drowsy. All too often it has been the medical attendant's intolerance of the bereaved's expression of anguish that has led to the immediate offer of a sedative so as to "keep everything and everybody quiet and calm."

As yet, there is no scientific evidence comparing the therapeutic effect of a sympathetic listener with a doctor who does little more than provide what is considered to be a suitable prescription. Nor do we know whether tranquilizers and antidepressants reduce the pain of grief or merely postpone it. Despite the scientific uncertainty, I suggest that the total denial of psychopharmacologic support in bereavement is both shortsighted and inhumane. Take, for example, the woman who has nursed her husband at home, with little outside help, throughout his terminal illness. The last few nights or more may well have been virtually sleepless, and she is totally exhausted with little or no mental and physical reserves with which to face her bereavement. The use of a bedtime hypnotic until, at least, after the funeral would seem to be reasonable. Other indications for the use of psychopharmacologic agents have been discussed in Goldberg et al. (1973). As always, of course, they should be used only as adjunctive therapy and not as substitutes for human care.

Postbereavement Family Support Service

Several studies confirm the potential pathogenic effect of major bereavement in adult life (Parkes 1965, Stein and Susser 1969, Parkes 1970, Birtchnell 1970a, b, c). Because of these reports, a postbereavement family support service was set up at St. Christopher's Hospice (London) some years ago in an endeavor to reduce postbereavement morbidity. First, it was necessary to identify those relatives at special risk and then to develop a service to reduce the incidence and degree of maladjustment. To this end, an eight-point questionnaire relating to the next-of-kin or "key person" was introduced based on the results of Parkes' Harvard Bereavement Study (Parkes 1975). It was hoped that, if completed by a member of the nursing staff shortly after a patient's death, it would be possible to predict the key person's state a year or so later. The eight questions were supplied with multiple-choice answers, which were scored from either 1 to 5 or 1 to 6. By adding the results, the investigators could arrive at an overall "predictive score." Each key person was then allocated to one of the following groups:

A. *Imperative need*
   These individuals are felt to be in great need of help, so much so that it would be unethical to withhold it. In practice, this means all those who have a high score on the eighth question—"How will key person cope?" This is, in effect, an intuitive assessment of the possible outcome.

B. *High risk*
   These have a predictive score of 18 or more and, unless thought to be antagonistic to follow-up, are randomly allocated either to an "experimental" or a "control" group, the control group being necessary for an objective assessment of the service.

C. *Low risk*
   Those with a predictive score of less than 18.

Follow-up visits were then arranged for the whole of group A and the experimental half of group B. The selection of the person to make the follow-up visit was discussed and where possible, the member of staff best known to the key person visited approximately two weeks after the bereavement. Help was given whenever possible, and further visits were arranged as considered necessary. Each month, visitors met with the social psychiatrist to discuss any problems that had arisen to plan further support and to consider ways of improving the service.

More than 1,500 questionnaires have now been completed. The distribution of the key persons is as follows:

Group A	82	(6%)
Group B	288	(19%)
Group C	1,145	(75%)

Of the 1,500 key persons, 227 (15 percent) have been visited, usually at least twice: that is, all group A and the experimental half of group B. With very few exceptions the visitors have been welcomed by the respondents and have been pleased with the results of their visits. Visitors see their main roles as: (1) providing continuity of contact with an understanding person—that is, someone with whom feelings about the bereavement can be expressed; (2) being a link to other forms of specialized help; (3) serving to assess the risk of suicidal behavior.

To evaluate the benefit of this service, some 40 to 50 key persons from each group were visited by an interviewer from the research unit 18 to 24 months after bereavement. The questions dealt with problems faced and help offered since bereavement, including any contact with St. Christopher's, and the key person's attitude to each source of help. The second half of the interview was a shortened version of the "Health Questionnaire" used to measure "outcome" in the Harvard Bereavement study (Parkes and Brown 1972).

Of the respondents, 104 were approached by the research interviewer. Twenty-five refused an interview, 18 could not be located, and 5 had died; the other 56 were interviewed for the project. The predictive score was not a highly reliable indicator of outcome 21 months after bereavement in that high-risk survivors were scattered fairly evenly along the y axis. However, the important practical question is not the correlation between predictive score and outcome but the reliability of the predictive questionnaire as a means of screening out a population, which will include those with a poor outcome. We must ask, therefore, what proportion of the respondents with poor outcome were identified as "high-risk" cases and what proportion were incorrectly classified as "low-risk." Taking a predictive score of 18 as our cutoff point for a "high-risk" case, we find that 13 of 17 (77 percent) of the poor outcome group were correctly designated as "high-risk" and 4 (23 percent) as "low-risk."

Further evidence for the predictive validity of the questionnaire relates to four respondents who committed suicide within two years after the death of their spouses. All four were found to have scored 18 or more on the predictive questionnaire. Modifications to the questionnaire are being made following a multivariate analysis of the findings to eventuate in a much sharper predictive instrument.

Terminal Care and Acute Grief

However helpful the family support service may prove to be, there is little doubt that a high standard of terminal care benefits not only the patient but also the relatives in their bereavement.

> I am very grateful for all you did for my mother. Although I am still very sad over her death, I get some comfort from the fact that she was in the very best place possible.
>
> * * * * * * * *.*
>
> We loved our sister and the knowledge of the loving care she received during her last dreadful illness will help sustain us in our grief.
>
> * * * * * * * * *
>
> You have proved by the peace with which you helped Doug on his way that death is not a thing to be feared. It gave us great comfort in our loss to know this.
>
> * * * * * * * * *
>
> Since my husband died last week my mind has been very confused. I miss him dreadfully and mixed with a certain guilty relief is an absolute horror at the disease and what it did to him. . . . The calm love you have shown us both over the past months has filled me with gratitude.

The last letter cited particularly emphasizes that good terminal care is not, nor could ever be, a means of erasing grief. The grief is still there, still hurts, still has to be coped with and worked through. Yet the memory of a dignified, peaceful death brings a tremendous "plus" factor into the total situation. What do I mean by good terminal care? First, I mean the kind of care in which every effort is made to overcome and keep at bay symptoms such as pain, nausea, constipation, anorexia, and breathlessness. Many of our patients require a narcotic analgesic regularly. Within the context of total patient care, this has been well documented (Saunders 1967, Lamerton 1973). I would emphasize, however, that it is possible for a patient to be free from pain and also fully alert when receiving drugs of this nature.

Second, I mean the kind of care in which patients are not isolated and enclosed in a mesh of negative thinking. Instead, they are respected as individuals, allowed to talk about their illness, allowed to work through to a positive acceptance of their death, and allowed to express their fears and anxieties concerning not so much their death as the manner of their dying. Will it be painful? Will I suffocate? How long will it be?

I also mean the kind of care in which the family is seen as part of the treatment unit; they, too, need to work through stages of denial, anger, and depression to a positive acceptance of the inevitable. Until they do, they can adversely affect the patient by maintaining and transferring unhelpful or negative attitudes. It is important to encourage them to continue to do things for the patient, such as tidying pillows; assisting, if necessary, at mealtimes; and joining in the activities that are arranged from time to time. In this connection, it is important for the staff not to "take" the patient from the family, not to become possessive and exclusive. To this end, it is imperative to have liberal visiting hours and to do away with restrictions such as "only two visitors to a patient" or "no children under 12."

A police sergeant, aged thirty-nine, was admitted to St. Christopher's with motor neuron disease. He was an inpatient for about two years and from time to time discussed his attitude toward illness with one of the doctors. He disliked phrases such as terminal or catastrophic illness; instead, he preferred "bring-together illness." When asked if he always saw this "bringing-together" happen, he replied, "Yes, I am a trained observer and

I've been here for 18 months. Patient and family, patient and staff, patient and patient—yes, it does happen" (Saunders 1973).

Because it takes time to help both patients and relatives reach the point where the illness can truly be called a "bring-together illness," we do not like having "bed and breakfast" patients, that is, patients who come in one day and die the next. However, since prognostication is an art and not a science, we shall always have a certain number of these extremely short-stay patients. But even here, there is quite a lot one can do, not the least being to assuage the guilt implied in such statements as "If we'd known it was going to be so short, we'd have kept him at home."

Conclusions

1. Psychopharmacologic agents have a definite, though limited, place in the management of acute grief.
2. Bereavement bears many similarities to an illness; it is certainly a state of ill health. A sensitive and reliable method for predicting the high-risk survivor is needed if we are to make the best use of our resources.
3. Meanwhile, it is important to develop a positive, almost aggressive, approach to the problems of terminal illness in order not only to help the patient to die in peace but also to give those who will be left behind the best possible support as they work through their grief.

References

Birtchnell, J. 1970a. "Recent Parent Death and Mental Illness." *British Journal of Psychiatry* 116:289.
―― 1970b. "Depression in Relation to Early and Recent Parental Death." *British Journal of Psychiatry* 116:299.
―― 1970c. "The Relationship Between Attempted Suicide, Depression and Parental Death." *British Journal of Psychiatry* 116:307.
Goldberg, I. K., S. Malitz and A. H. Kutscher, eds. 1973. *Psychopharmacologic Agents for the Terminally Ill and Bereaved*, New York: Columbia University Press.
Kübler-Ross, E. 1973. "On the Use of Psychopharmacologic Agents for the Dying Patient and the Bereaved." In I. K. Goldberg, et al., eds.

Psychopharmacologic Agents for the Terminally Ill and Bereaved, New York: Columbia University Press.

Lamerton, R. C. 1973. *Care of the Dying*. London: Priory Press.

Parkes, C. M. 1965. "Bereavement and Mental Illness." *British Journal of Medical Psychology* 38:1.

―――― 1970. "The Psychosomatic Effects of Bereavement." In O. W. Hill, ed. *Modern Trends in Psychosomatic Medicine* vol. 20. London: Butterworth.

―――― 1972. *Bereavement: Studies of Grief in Adult Life*. London: Tavistock.

Parkes, C. M. 1975. "Unexpected and Untimely Bereavement: A Statistical Study of Young Boston Widows and Widowers." In B. Schoenberg et al., eds. *Bereavement: Its Psychosocial Aspects*. New York: Columbia University Press.

Parkes, C. M. and R. J. Brown. 1972. "Health After Bereavement: A Controlled Study of Young Boston Widows and Widowers." *Psychosomatic Medicine* 34:449.

Saunders, C. M. S. 1967. *The Management of Terminal Illness*. London: Hospital Medicine Publications.

―――― 1973. "A Death in the Family: A Professional View." *British Medical Journal* 1:30.

Stein, Z. and M. Susser. 1969. "Widowhood and Mental Illness." *British Journal of Medicine* 23:106.

21.
PSYCHOPHARMACOLOGIC TREATMENT OF BEREAVEMENT

ROBERT KELLNER, RICHARD T. RADA, AND WALTER W. WINSLOW

No adequate research has been done on the psychopharmacologic treatment of the bereaved. Views apparently differ about the value of pharmacotherapy in bereavement, whether it is necessary or whether it is even desirable.

Only a few would agree today with Benjamin Rush's advice that the best management of grief is a prescription of "liberal doses of opium" (1835). An indication of how drug treatment is regarded by most authors is the fact that the *Cumulative Index Medicus* does not list a single title on the pharmacotherapy of the bereaved. Moreover, in several articles on the management of bereavement or on the factors influencing the outcome of bereavement, pharmacotherapy is not mentioned at all (Kalish 1970, Kutscher and Goldberg 1973, Kutscher and Kutscher 1971, Maddison and Walker 1967, McCourt et al. 1976, Sarmousakis 1966) or is mentioned only in passing. For example, Patterson (1969) merely mentions in a case history that the patient was treated with an antidepressant. Saunders (1973) mentions briefly that the attitudes of the professionals are more important than just giving "sympathy and sedatives," and a few others make brief recommendations: Gramlich (1968) mentions that tranquilizing or antidepressant drugs can be used depending on the target symptoms. Rees (1973) mentions that at times the judicious use of tranquilizers, antidepressants, and analgesics will suffice. Bowen (1973) recommends antianxiety and antidepressant drugs "when any abnormal development occurs." He comments that it has sometimes been suggested "that to give antidepressants to someone bereaved is to run against the course of nature," and he calls this "an argument perhaps analogous to that once used to justify the withholding of anesthesia in childbirth." An exception, and perhaps a reversal of this trend, was evident among the contributors to a text on the drug treatment for the terminally ill and the bereaved (Goldberg et al. 1973).

Drugs are frequently prescribed for the bereaved. Parkes (1972), Parkes and Brown (1972), and Ferguson (1973) found an increased use of tranquilizers by the bereaved. Yet there is a remarkable lack of research in pharmacotherapy of the bereaved. The reason for this is unclear. We discussed this topic with several psychopharmacologists, seeking their opinion about why this field had not been researched. The answers tended to vary somewhat, but views were expressed to the effect that bereavement is not an appropriate topic for psychopharmacologic research, because bereavement is a normal reaction that is only short-lived and not in the realm of the psychiatrist. Other views indicated that mourning does not differ essentially from other distress and other losses and that general principles of psychopharmacology would apply here as they do in other kinds of distress. A few expressed the view that recently bereaved people form only a small proportion of the psychiatric clinic population and thus are not easily accessible to the researcher. Two researchers voiced reluctance based on scruples because of their respect for the grief that bereaved people experience and said that they were hesitant to include bereaved people in experiments in therapeutics (unpublished personal communications).

It is conceivable that psychopharmacologic treatment of a recently bereaved person is harmful. Psychiatrists and psychologists have expressed views to the effect that interference with the process of mourning might lead to more serious disturbance later. Freud (1917) believed that interference with grieving can be harmful. Deutsch (1937) believed that grief that is not adequately expressed at the time will be expressed later in a pathologic form. Similar views have been voiced by others (Lindemann 1944, Maddison and Raphael 1973, Paul and Grosser 1965, Volkan and Showalter 1968). Parkes (1964) believes that those who fail to express their distress within the first week or two of bereavement are more likely than others to be disturbed later. He found that "delayed reactions" were more often found in psychiatric patients who were bereaved than in unselected bereaved people who were not psychiatric patients. This raises the possibility that an energetic drug treatment might merely delay grieving or may even contribute to the development of a subsequent psychiatric illness. Maddison and Viola (1968) and Maddison and Raphael (1973) found in a retrospective study of widows that the taking of psychotropic drugs was related to poor outcome. However, drug treatment may not have been the cause of the poor outcome; it seems likely that the psychotropic drugs were prescribed for widows who were unusually distressed or were not making an adequate recovery.

Several authors caution against the use of psychotropic drugs. Kübler-Ross (1973) believes that "to sedate the bereaved quickly in order to keep their anguish from others is very harmful from a therapeutic point of view: it only postpones expression of anger and guilt and thus prolongs grief," and she cautions that psychopharmacologic agents should always and only be used as adjunctive therapy and not as substitutes for human care. Wiener (1973) believes that "psychopharmacologic agents should be used to facilitate the expression of feeling or when the suffering of bereavement is so intense or pathological that the normal process of bereavement and expression of feeling is paralyzed." Similarly, Arkin (1973) believes that one should not attempt to avert or suppress grief but administer only those drugs and in such quantities that grief does not become excessively disorganizing and destructive to the person. Parkes (1972) believes that drugs do not frequently have a damaging effect in bereavement, that "their use is so widespread that any serious consequences would have probably become apparent already if they were at all frequent," but recommends that until their effects have been properly assessed they should be used with caution.

Another possible hazard of drug treatment of the bereaved is the abuse of or addiction to the prescribed drugs. This is suggested by evidence of increased use of psychotropic drugs (Parkes 1971) and increased risk of alcohol addiction in the bereaved. In one study of 150 bereaved psychiatric patients, 13 had become chronic alcoholics (Parkes 1972). In a study of widows in Boston (Parkes and Brown 1972) and another study of widows in London (Parkes 1971) 38 percent and 31 percent, respectively, were drinking more alcohol and smoking more after the bereavement than before. Clayton et al. (1968) found that social drinkers did not have a tendency to increase the amount of alcohol after bereavement, but heavy drinkers and alcoholics tended to do so. However, Parkes (1965) reports relapse of alcoholics after bereavement, and the present authors have observed patients who were social drinkers before bereavement who became heavy drinkers later. One of our patients, a sixty-three-year-old widower whose wife died of cancer, stated: "We were sweethearts for forty years, the only time I can forget her is when I drink." Several admissions to psychiatric hospitals interrupted his drinking temporarily. He died one and a half years later, at which time he was drinking on the average a pint of whisky a day. The increased mortality of the bereaved that has been found by several investigators is probably caused in part by increased alcohol consumption, drugs, and self-neglect (Epstein et al. 1968). Although a definite increase of alcohol consumption has been found in bereaved people, only a small proportion of the bereaved apparently become alcoholics.

Krant (1975) mentions that an excessive use of psychotropic drugs has been reported after bereavement. However, the danger of addiction to psychotropic drugs appears to be smaller than the risk of alcoholism. In Parkes' study of forty-four unselected lonely widows (1971), three quarters had consulted a general practitioner during the first six months of bereavement, thirteen of these were treated with sedatives or tranquilizers, but only three were still taking them a year to eighteen months later, and all three had been taking drugs before bereavement. It could be argued that treatment with psychotropic drugs might lessen the risk of psychiatric consequences, including alcoholism, but this is not certain.

In the absence of prospective controlled studies of pharmacotherapy of the bereaved, we have based our recommendations on our experiences of the treatment of the bereaved and have tried to apply principles of psychopharmacology derived from research with psychiatric patients. When discussing psychopharmacologic treatment, we tried, in accord with the view of others (Maddison and Raphael 1973, Parkes 1965, Wahl 1970), to distinguish between the period of normal grief and psychiatric complications that can occur, although this distinction is arbitrary and often difficult to make.

Mourning

We believe with other investigators (Kübler-Ross 1973, Maddison and Raphael 1973, Parkes 1964, Schmale 1973, Wiener 1973) that pharmacotherapy during the mourning phase should be used with caution, and we do not routinely advise a bereaved person to take psychotropic drugs to relieve distress. Ferguson (1973) found that more than one third of the widows she studied did not require tranquilizers. Moreover, bereaved persons who are not severely distressed and request medication should be advised to try to avoid taking drugs because of the doubtful benefits and the risks of unwanted effects. They should be told that psychotropic drugs will not abolish the void, the painful emptiness or the feeling of loss—that all they can do is partially relieve some of the symptoms. However, if the distress is unusually severe or substantially interferes with continuing family functions (such as a widow who has become unable to care adequately for her small children) or with essential employment, psychotropic drugs should be prescribed as in other severe adjustment reactions. Under these circumstances the bereaved may be encouraged to take drugs as a temporary crutch, albeit a necessary one, to facilitate coping with the crisis.

Which Drugs To Choose

The drugs chosen will depend on the kind of distress the bereaved person experiences. The most common symptoms during the mourning phase are depression, anxiety, insomnia, and psychophysiologic symptoms. Increased presence of depressive symptoms has been found in several studies. Parkes (1972) regards depression as so common that absence of depression after bereavement is more abnormal than its presence. Several investigators have reported an increased prevalence of anxiety. Clayton and her colleagues (1968) found that more than one third of the bereaved had anxiety attacks. Roth (1959) found phobic aversion of leaving familiar surroundings in bereaved people. Crisp and Priest (1972) found increased distress, including anxiety and depression as measured by the Middlesex Health Questionnaire. Marris (1958) found that all widows in his study reported either depression or anxiety, whereas Yamamoto et al. (1969) found anxiety or depression in 85 percent of widows. Several investigators have reported that anxiety and depression tend to occur together in psychiatric non-psychotic patients (Kellner et al. 1972, McNair and Lorr 1964, Rickels 1968), and apparently a similar relationship of anxiety to depression exists also in the bereaved.

Minor tranquilizers may become necessary during the mourning phase. Ferguson (1973) found that this need is apparently influenced by several factors, including the personality of the bereaved and the relationship of the bereaved to the lost person. A few bereaved persons experience severe anxiety and tension, particularly after the initial shock has passed, and they have to face emotional and economic adjustment and other problems of living without the loved one. In the case of a bereaved spouse this can often induce fear: a thirty-five-year-old woman with four children, who had not worked since she was nineteen, lost her husband in an accident, and she described her feelings as follows: "I felt I was expected to walk, just having lost both legs; it was terrifying." For the anxiety and tension that occur in these situations minor tranquilizers are usually adequate. The safest are the benzodiazepines (Kellner 1975a) (chlordiazepoxide, diazepam, oxazepam, clorazepate). In controlled studies, the benzodiazepines have been found to be either as effective as or more effective than major tranquilizers, other minor tranquilizers, or barbiturates (Kellner et al. 1974).

If the patient has suffered from incapacitating or severe anxiety for a long time, psychotropic drugs may produce a vacation from fear and may interrupt a vicious cycle such as anxiety's contributing to poor work performance, leading to more anxiety, and so on. Initially, the tranquilizer should be taken regularly and in doses that are adequate to relieve all or most of the anxiety. About three to four weeks after the patient's anxiety has been controlled, the weaning process should begin. The medication can be withdrawn gradually by reducing the dose or by advising the patient to take the drug intermittently; the latter regimen has the advantage that medication is taken only on the day when the patient feels distressed and unnecessary medication is not taken on days when the patient does not feel anxious. The severity of anxiety tends to fluctuate markedly in most patients, particularly during recovery. Remissions can last from a few hours to several weeks, and recurrences appear to be almost as severe as the initial attack but are usually of shorter duration. In most patients recurrences become less frequent and eventually cease. The patient's knowledge that the dose can be self-adjusted (which in practice many patients do regardless of the physician's instructions) may give the patient the added security that anxiety can be relieved if the distress becomes excessive. Later, the patient may resume medication only at times of recurrence of anxiety and discontinue it when the symptoms wane. There are some patients who suffer from anxiety for a long period and may need regular antianxiety medication to control disabling symptoms (Kellner 1975a).

When anxiety and depression coexist or when the adjustment reaction is manifested largely by depression, antianxiety medications may be tried first, largely because of their rapid onset of action.

In many patients who are anxious and depressed, the relief of anxiety alone will also lead to relief of depression, as though when anxiety and tensions are relieved, unhappiness and misery lessen too (Kellner 1975a, Kellner et al. 1974). If, after all anxiety has been relieved, the patient is still markedly depressed, then the diagnosis and the treatment should be reconsidered. If the patient reports feeling worse after anxiety is relieved or not feeling anxious any longer but feeling more depressed, antidepressant drugs should be considered. The patient may have symptoms of an early type of "endogenous" depression, or if treated with a benzodiazepine, it may be a rare idiosyncratic side effect of the benzodiazepine (Hall and Jaffe 1972, Ryan et al. 1968).

There is no conclusive research evidence that would indicate that one benzodiazepine is more effective than another, except perhaps for the treatment of hostility. Anger and manifest hostility to others are common during mourning. Hostility in bereavement was reported by Lindemann (1944); Marris (1958) found that some degree of irritability and anger is usual, and Peretz (1970) mentions overt or disguised hostility as one of the reactions to loss. Stern et al. (1951) found irrational hostility in old people, and anger was admitted by most widows in Parkes' London study (1971). Hostility alone seldom requires treatment in the bereaved. However, if it appears that hostility becomes more apparent after treatment with one of the older benzodiazepines, it is worth trying to change the treatment to oxazepam because it appears to be less likely to induce hostility and has perhaps greater antihostility effects (DiMascio et al. 1969, Gardos et al. 1968, Kellner 1975a, Shader 1971).

Some antipsychotic drugs, for example, thioridazine and chlorpromazine, have been successfully used both in the treatment of anxiety and in anxiety-depression (Overall and Henry 1973, Overall et al. 1964, Raskin 1974). In view of the long term risks of tardive dyskinesia, they should not be used in the treatment of bereavement.

The extent to which tricyclic drugs have a mood-elevating effect during mourning is uncertain. Some authors recommend their use if the depression is severe (Hollister 1973, Rees 1973). They are usually the treatment of first choice if bereavement is complicated by the onset of a psychotic depression. In view of their antidepressant and antianxiety effects, safety, and absence of tolerance, they can be the drug of first choice if the patient can tolerate their side effects (Covi et al. 1974). Their use, either alone or in combination with other drugs, is described below.

Several authors have reported that sleep disturbances are common after bereavement. Marris (1958) reported insomnia as a common symptom in widows. Parkes (1971) found that 75 percent of unselected bereaved complained of insomnia, and Clayton et al. (1968) found sleep disturbance in 85 percent. Prolonged insomnia, particularly if the patient is worried about it, can establish a vicious cycle. The patient gets more concerned about not being able to sleep, fears not being able to sleep, and does not relax adequately. Moreover, prolonged sleeplessness may make the patient feel lethargic during the day and less able to cope with everyday problems. The prescribing of a hypnotic for a short time in these cases may be indicated (Arkin 1973, Hollister 1973). Flurazepam (Dalmane), temazepam (Restoril), and triazolam (Halcion) are benzodiazepine hypnotics that are marketed in the United States at present; they are decidedly safer than other classes of hypnotics. The risk, even with a safe hypnotic, is the development of tolerance and inhabituation. Patients who take hypnotics regularly were found not to sleep any longer, nor did they fall asleep more quickly than insomniacs who were not taking hypnotics (Johns et al. 1970). After having slept several consecutive nights, the patient should be advised to reduce the amount being taken. The patient should be told to try to fall asleep without the hypnotic but to leave the prescribed number of tablets for one night (not the whole bottle) at the bedside. If the patient does not fall asleep, only a part of the dose should be taken first, and if the patient is still awake about half an hour later, the remainder should be taken. Some nights the patient will fall asleep without any night sedation or with having taken only part of the dose. By this method, weaning is likely to be more rapid than when the patient takes hypnotics regularly. Clift (1972) found that when a physician frequently reviewed the prescription and offered encouraging advice about sleeping without hypnotics, the amount of hypnotics taken and the proportion of patients who were still taking hypnotics after one year were substantially reduced, as compared with patients who were treated by physicians who prescribed hypnotics in a traditional way.

Psychiatric Complications of Bereavement

Bereavement can have various complications. The danger of alcholism has been described. Suicide rates are increased (Bunch 1972, Rushing 1968), particularly in alcoholics (Murphy and Robins 1967). Lindemann (1944) reported a greater incidence of psychosomatic disorders. Bereaved people have a greater mortality than people who have not been bereaved (Cox and Ford 1964, Kraus and Lilienfeld 1959, Parkes et al. 1969, Rees and Lutkins 1967, Young et al. 1963). Psychiatric illness has been found more common in the bereaved than in the nonbereaved controls (Parkes 1964, Parkes and Brown 1972). Stein and Susser (1969) found that widows are more likely to enter psychiatric care for the first time than women of the same age who have not been bereaved. There is an increase in psychiatric hospitalizations for the bereaved (Parkes 1964, Pugh and MacMahon 1962, Stein and Susser 1969). Clayton (1979) has reviewed the literature on conjugal bereavement.

Psychosis appears to be a rare consequence of bereavement; both mania and schizophrenia are rare sequels (Parkes 1965). The occurrence of several cases of "endogenous" depression after bereavement has been described by Muller-Fahlbusch (1971), but Anderson, in his earlier studies, found only 4 percent of the psychiatric diagnoses after bereavement were "anergic" depressions (1949).

There is no clearcut dividing line between the almost inevitable adjustment reaction during mourning and the beginning of a depression, which could be regarded as a psychiatric complication. The duration, intensity, and the form of mourning differ a great deal from one person to another. It seems logical to prescribe psychotropic drugs when the distress seems excessive or incapacitating and the patient has not responded adequately to psychotherapy. The clinical picture is usually that of an adjustment disorder with depressed mood (or "reactive" depression) (Parkes 1965), and the pharmacotherapy is the same as that described above under the management of mourning when anxiety and depression coexist. Although only a small proportion of the bereaved will experience a psychotic depressive reaction, it is important to be alert for its early symptoms. The diagnostic approach is the same as in distinguishing between exogenous and endogenous depressions (neurotic and psychotic depressions); the early signs and symptoms that tend to herald the "physiologic shift" include an increase in psychomotor retardation, guilt and self-accusation, greater symptom severity in the morning, onset of suicidal ruminations, failure to react to changes in the environment (such as to good or bad news), and an increase in vegetative symptoms, particularly loss of appetite and weight loss. If a psychotic depressive reaction occurs or if an early endogenous component is suspected, energetic treatment with tricyclic antidepressants in adequate doses is indicated. The suicide risk must be carefully assessed. If a danger of suicide appears to be present and there is inadequate supervision of the patient at home, hospitalization should be considered. Many psychiatrists believe that, when anxiety and depression coexist and the response to antidepressants alone does not relieve anxiety, a combination of an antianxiety drug and an antidepressant drug should be tried (Merlis 1973). This combination has a logical appeal, but there is no conclusive evidence that the effects of this combination are superior to those of the individual drugs (Kellner 1970, Kellner 1975a). The decision to use this combination of drugs should be made only after the response to both antidepressants and antianxiety drugs alone was found to be inadequate. One should determine the optimal dosage for each drug separately rather than prescribe one tablet with the two drugs combined in a fixed ratio.

The monoamine oxidase inhibitors have proven antidepressant effects in neurotic depression and in anxiety (Sheehan et al. 1980). In view of the risks of interactions with other drugs and with foods with high tyramine content, they should be used only if the depression fails to respond to other treatments.

Several other drugs have been found to have an antidepressant effect in endogenous depression. The research evidence at present is not conclusive enough to recommend their use in uncomplicated depression. The pharmacotherapy of the less frequent psychiatric and psychosomatic complications of bereavement is outside the scope of the present paper.

In summary, the physician's role in bereavement should be primarily that of a counselor and psychotherapist. His or her other role is to be alert to the psychiatric and psychosomatic complications of bereavement. Bereavement in itself is not an indication for psychopharmacologic treatment although it may have an important role to play if the distress is unbearable or incapacitating, if psychiatric or psychosomatic complications occur, and if the response to psychotherapy is inadequate.

References

Anderson, C. 1949. "Aspects of Pathological Grief and Mourning." *International Journal of Psycho-Analysis* 30:40.

Arkin, A. M. 1973. "The Use of Medications in the Management of the Dying Patient and the Bereaved." In I. K. Goldberg et al., eds. (1973): 72–76.

Bowen, A. 1973. "The Psychiatric Aspects of Bereavement." *Practitioner* 210:127.

Bunch, J. 1972. "Recent Bereavement in Relation to Suicide." *Journal of Psychosomatic Research* 16:361.

Clayton, P. J. 1979. "The Sequaelae and Nonsequelae of Conjugal Bereavement." *American Journal of Psychiatry* 136:1530.

Clayton, P., L. Desmarais, and G. Winokur 1968. "A Study of Normal Bereavement." *American Journal of Psychiatry* 125:168.

Clift, A. D. 1972. "Factors Leading to Dependence on Hypnotic Drugs." *British Medical Journal* 3:614.

Covi, L., R. S. Lipman, L. R. Derogatis, et al. 1974. "Drugs and Group Psychotherapy in Neurotic Depression." *American Journal of Psychiatry* 131:191.

Cox, P. R. and J. R. Ford, 1964. "The Mortality of Widows Shortly After Widowhood." *Lancet* 1:163.

Crisp, A. H. and R. G. Priest 1972. "Psychoneurotic Status During the Year Following Bereavement." *Journal of Psychosomatic Research* 16:351.

Deutsch, H. 1937. "Absence of Grief." *Psychoanalytic Quarterly* 6:12.

DiMascio, A., R. I. Shader and J. Hermatz 1969. "Psychotropic Drugs and Induced Hostility." *Psychosomatics* 10:46.

Epstein, G., L. Weitz, H. Roback, and E. McKee 1968. "A Research on Bereavement. A Selective and Critical Review." *Comprehensive Psychiatry* 16:537.

Ferguson, T. 1973. "Decision-Making and Tranquilizers in Widowhood." In I. K. Goldberg et al., eds. (1973):225–34.

Freud, S. 1957. "Mourning and Melancholia (1917)." *Complete Works*, Standard Edition, vol 19. London: Hogarth Press.

Gardos, G., A. DiMascio, C. Salzman, and R. I. Shader. 1968. "Differential Actions of Chlordiazepoxide and Oxazepam on Hostility." *Archives of General Psychiatry* 18:757.
Goldberg, I. K., S. Malitz, and A. H. Kutscher. 1973. *Psychopharmacologic Agents for the Terminally Ill and Bereaved*. New York: Columbia University Press.
Gramlich, E. P. 1968. "Recognition and Management of Grief in Elderly Patients." *Geriatrics* (July) 23:87–92.
Hall, R. C. and J. R. Joffe. 1972. "Aberrant Response to Diazepam: A New Syndrome." *American Journal of Psychiatry* 129:738.
Hollister, L. E. 1973. "Psychotherapeutic Drugs in the Dying and Bereaved." In I. K. Goldberg et al., eds. (1973):65–71.
Johns, M. W. et al. 1970. "Sleep Habits and Symptoms in Male Medical and Surgical Patients." *British Medical Journal* 2:509.
Kalish, R. A. 1970. "Loss and Grief. A Selected Bibliography." In B. B. Schoenberg et al., eds. (1970):373–84.
Kellner, R. 1970. "Drugs, Diagnoses and Outcome of Drug Trials with Neurotic Patients. A Survey." *Journal of Nerve and Mental Disorders* 151:85.
Kellner, R. 1975. "The Clinical Pharmacology of Anxiety." In M. Marshall, ed. *Clinical Psychopharmacology 1975*. New York: Jason Aaronson.
Kellner, R., G. M. Simpson, and W. W. Winslow. 1972. "The Relationship of Depressive Neurosis to Anxiety and Somatic Symptoms." *Psychosomatics* 13:358.
Kellner, R., W. W., Winslow, and R. Rada. 1974. "The Pharmacotherapy of Anxiety and Depressive Neurosis." *Medical World News* (October).
Krant, M. J. 1975. "A Death in the Family." *Journal of the American Medical Association* 231:195.
Kraus, A. S. and A. M. Lilienfeld. 1959. "Some Epidemiologic Aspects of the High Mortality Rate in the Young Widowed Group." *Journal of Chronic Diseases* 10:207.
Kübler-Ross, E. 1973. "On the Use of Psychopharmacologic Agents for the Dying Patient and the Bereaved." In I. K. Goldberg et al., eds. (1973):3–6.
Kutscher, A. H. and M. R. Goldberg. 1973. *Caring for the Dying Patient and His Family*. New York: Health Sciences Publishing Corp.
Kutscher, A. H. and L. G. Kutscher, eds. 1971. *For the Bereaved*. New York: Frederick Fell.
Lindemann, E. 1944. "Symptomatology and Management of Acute Grief." *American Journal of Psychiatry* 101:141.
Maddison, D. and B. Raphael. 1973. "Normal Bereavement as an Illness Requiring Care: Psychopharmacological Approaches." In I. K. Goldberg, et al., eds (1973):235–48.
Maddison, D. and A. Viola. 1968. "The Health of Widows in the Year Following Bereavement." *Journal of Psychosomatic Research* 12:297.
Maddison, D. and W. L. Walker. 1967. "Factors Affecting the Outcome of Conjugal Bereavement." *British Journal of Psychiatry* 113:1057.

Marris, P. 1958. *Widows and Their Families* London: Routledge.
McCourt, W. F., R. D. Barnett, J. Brennen, and A. Becker 1976. "We Help Each Other: Primary Prevention for the Widowed." *American Journal of Psychiatry* 133:98.
McNair, D. M. and M. Lorr, 1964. "An Analysis of Mood in Neurotics." *Journal of Abnormal Social Psychology* 69:620.
Merlis, S. 1973. "Antianxiety Agents in the Management of the Bereaved." In I. K. Goldberg et al, eds. (1973):165–70.
Muller-Fahlbusch, H. 1971. "Endogene Depressive Phasen nach dem Tode eines Angehorigen." *Nervenarzt* 42:426.
Murphy, G. E. and E. Robins. 1967. "Social Factors in Suicide." *Journal of the American Medical Association* 199:303.
Overall, J. E. and B. W. Henry. 1973. "Decisions About Drug Therapy. Selection of Treatment for Psychiatric Inpatients." *Archives of General Psychiatry* 28:81.
Overall J. E., L. E. Hollister, F. Meyer, I. Kimbell, Jr., and J. Shelton. 1964. "Imipramine and Thioridazine in Depressed and Schizophrenic Patients." *Journal of the American Medical Association* 189:605.
Parkes, C. M. 1964. "Recent Bereavement as a Cause of Mental Illness." *British Journal of Psychiatry* 110:198.
Parkes, C. M. 1965a. "Bereavement and Mental Illness. Part 1. A Clinical Study of the Grief of Bereaved Psychiatric Patients." *British Journal of Medical Psychology* 38:1.
Parkes, C. M. 1965b. "Bereavement and Mental Illness. Part 2. A Classification of Bereavement Reactions." *British Journal of Medical Psychology* 38:13.
Parkes, C. M. 1971. "The First Year of Bereavement: A Longitudinal Study of the Reaction of London Widows to the Death of Their Husbands." *Psychiatry* 33:444.
Parkes, C. M. 1972. *Bereavement. Studies of Grief in Adult Life* New York: International Universities Press, Inc.
Parkes, C. M., B. Benjamin, and R. G. Fitzgerald. 1969. "Broken Heart: A Statistical Study of Increased Mortality Among Widowers." *British Medical Journal* 1:740.
Parkes, C. M. and R. J. Brown. 1972. "Health After Bereavement: A Controlled Study of Young Boston Widows and Widowers." *Psychosomatic Medicine* 34:449.
Patterson, R. D. 1969. "Grief and Depression in Old People." *Maryland Medical Journal* 18:75.
Paul, N. L. and G. H. Grosser. 1965. "Operational Mourning and Its Role in Conjoint Therapy." *Community Mental Health Journal* 1:339.
Peretz, D. 1970. "Development, Object-relationships, and Loss." In B. B. Schoenberg et al, eds. (1970):3–19.
Pugh, T. F. and B. MacMahon. 1962. *Epidemiologic Findings in U.S. Mental Hospital Data* Boston: Little, Brown.
Raskin, A. 1974. "A Guide for Drug Use in Depressive Disorders." *American Journal of Psychiatry* 131:181.

Rees, W. D. 1973. "Bereavement and Illness." In I. K. Goldberg et al, eds. 1973:264–69.
Rees, W. D. and S. G. Lutkins. 1967. "Mortality of Bereavement." *British Medical Journal* 4:13–16.
Rickels, K. 1968. "Drug Use in Outpatient Treatment. Supplement." *American Journal of Psychiatry* 124:20.
Roth, M. 1959. "The Phobic-Anxiety/Depersonalization Syndrome." *Proceeding of the Royal Society of Medicine* 52:587.
Rush, B. 1835. *Medical Inquiries and Observations upon the Diseases of the Mind.* Philadelphia: Grigg and Elliott.
Rushing, W. A. 1968. "Individual Behavior and Suicide." In J. P. Gibbs, eds, *Suicide.* New York: Harper & Row.
Ryan, H. F., F. B. Merrill, G. E. Scott, et al. 1968. "Increase in Suicidal Thoughts and Tendencies: Association with Diazepam Therapy." *Journal of the American Medical Association* 203:1137.
Sarmousakis, G. 1966. "Prevention of Depression in Relatives of Terminal Patients." *Delaware Medical Journal* 38:315.
Saunders, C. 1973. "A Death in the Family: A Professional View." *British Medical Journal* 1:30.
Schmale, A. H., Jr. 1973. "Normal Grief Is Not a Disease." In I. K. Goldberg et al., eds. (1973): pp. 257–63,
Schoenberg, B. B. et al., eds. 1970. *Loss and Grief: Psychological Management in Medical Practice.* New York: Columbia University Press.
Shader, R. I. 1971. "Drugs in the Management of Anxiety." *Current Psychiatric Therapeutics* 11:81.
Sheehan, D. V., J. Ballenger, and G. Jacobsen. 1980. "Treatmnt of Endogenous Anxiety with Phobia, Hysterical, and Hypochondriacal Symptoms." *Archives of General Psychiatry* 37:51–59.
Stein, Z. and M. W. Susser. 1969. "Widowhood and Mental Illness." *British Journal of Preventive & Social Medicine* 23:106.
Stern, K., G. M. Williams, and M. Prados. 1951. "Grief Reactions in Later Life." *American Journal of Psychiatry* 108:289.
Volkan, V. and C. R. Showalter. 1968. "Known Object Loss, Disturbance in Reality Testing and Grief Work as a Method of Brief Psychotherapy." *Psychiatric Quarterly* 42:358.
Wahl, C. 1970. "The Differential Diagnosis of Normal and Neurotic Grief Following Bereavement." *Archives of the Foundation of Thanatology* 1:137.
Wiener, A. 1973. "The Use of Psychopharmacologic Agents in the Management of the Bereaved." In I. K. Goldberg et al., eds. (1973):249–25.
Yamamoto, T., K. Okonogi, T. Iwasaki, and S. Yoshimura. 1969. "Mourning in Japan." *American Journal of Psychiatry* 125:74.
Young, M., B. Benjamin, and C. Wallis. 1963. "Mortality of Widowers." *Lancet* 2:454.

22.
TRICYCLIC ANTIDEPRESSANTS IN THE TREATMENT OF DEPRESSION IN CONJUGAL BEREAVEMENT: A CONTROLLED STUDY

Philip R. Muskin and Arthur Rifkin

Is grief a "normal" process or is it an illness? We recognize that someone who mourns appears sad, cries, suffers, and cannot enjoy life. Further, we commonly associate mourning with symptoms of insomnia, loss of appetite with weight loss, fatigue, and somatic complaints such as headaches, dizziness, or blurred vision. Part of grief, we now acknowledge, are feelings of not having done enough, self-blame for the death, anger toward doctors and others who cared for the deceased, or anger at the person for dying. Thus, mourners appear to be depressed, with many features of their suffering similar to those of patients with diagnosed affective illness.

Freud (1917) noted the similarity between mourning and the pathological state of melancholia, with the essential difference that the mourner had no loss of self-regard, the world had been "impoverished," while the melancholic suffered from a loss of self-esteem, and the ego was impoverished. Freud does not aver that mourning and melancholia have a causal relationship but asserts that some individuals who do not mourn suffer melancholia instead. Our questions are: What is the best treatment, if any, for the depression commonly seen during bereavement? What is pathological grief? What should we do about it?

Is grief normal? Lindemann (1944) and Parkes (1970) observed the course and clinical picture of grief. As early studies of mourning, their writings are descriptively rich, but there is little attention devoted to what normal grief is, as opposed to a pathological reaction. Lindemann does assert that any inhibition or delay of grief leads to a pathological response—a common belief that has not been proved. Parkes details widows' responses over time, but he makes no attempt to separate normal grief from the pathological (or potentially so). Clayton et al. (1968) show that three symptoms appear commonly in early mourning: depressed mood (87 percent), sleep disturbances (85 percent), and crying (79 percent). These symptoms usually diminished greatly during the first four months of mourning. Suicidal thoughts, loss of interest in activities, and self-condemnation were not frequent and had a relatively stable rate of occurrence over time. Improvement began at about six to ten weeks, which is comparable to Lindemann's work. Other common symptoms observed by Clayton and her colleagues were difficulty concentrating (47 percent), loss of interest in the television or news (42 percent), anxiety attacks (36 percent), irritability (36 percent), and anorexia and weight loss (49 percent). About one third of the mourners used sedative drugs. No one began to use alcohol for the first time during the bereavement period, but heavy drinkers and alcoholics increased their drinking.

Parkes notes several stages of grief in the widows he observed for one year:

1. Numbness. Though usually transient, it lasted as little as one day but was observed at two years in some. Panic attacks, outbursts of anger, tearfulness, or restlessness were all observed during the initial phase of grief.

2. Yearning or protest. This phase seemed to last a long time, even being observed at the anniversary of the death. Widows were preoccupied with thoughts of the deceased, cried, and were restless. He found almost half had hallucinations at some time during the first month following the death of their husband, which they all recognized as hallucinations (Clayton's work reveals only a 3 percent incidence).

3. Disorganization. Apathy and aimlessness predominate. It was impossible to judge the duration of this phase, because two thirds of the sample were still felt to be in this phase at the end of the year.

4. A final phase in which the widow reorganizes and integrates the loss into her life comes at varying times, dependent on each individual's situation.

Overall, Parkes found that 14 percent of the widows, the year after their loss, were poorly adjusted, depressed, and still grieving, and 68 percent were either intermittently depressed or had struck a tenuous balance that could be easily upset. At one month after the loss of their spouses, in the survey by Clayton et al., 35 percent were diagnosed as definitely or probably depressed by the criteria of Feighner et al. (1972). When these depressed widows and widowers were compared with those not diagnosed as depressed, no differences could be found in terms of age, socioeconomic status, religion, sex, prior treatment for depression, current personality diagnosis, or family history of affective disorder or alcoholism. At follow-up 13 months after the death of the spouse, Bornstein et al. (1973) found that 17 percent were still diagnosed as depressed, which compares to Parkes' findings (14 percent). Of the original 38 with the diagnosis of depression at one month, 12 (32 percent) were still depressed one year later. Three became depressed at four months and were still depressed at 13 months. Only one woman had a delayed onset of depression 13 months after the loss. From these data, it is clear that 13.6 percent of the entire sample was depressed for the greater portion of the first year following the loss of a spouse and that the only predictor, but a clearly powerful one, of who would be depressed at one year was the diagnosis of depression at one month. In a replication study, Clayton has found that severe grief is associated with a history of depression and thus offers support to the contention that such grief reactions are a type of depression that is not necessarily a "normal" process (1978). The work of Clayton et al. (1972) shows there is a rather substantial subgroup of individuals who, during conjugal bereavement, suffer from a clearly pathological condition—depression severe enough to meet the rigorous criteria of Feighner et al.

Pathological grief has been the focus of many workers, including Lindemann (1944), Greenblatt (1978), and Burgess (1976). Wahl (1970) lists several features diagnostic of pathological grief, including excessive and protracted grief, inability to deal with the opposing feelings of anger at and love for the deceased, development of symptoms similar to the deceased, irrational despair, severe feelings of hopelessness and loss of identity, impaired self esteem, self-blame for the death, protracted apathy, irritability, or hyperactivity without appropriate affect. It is noteworthy that the majority of these features are also diagnostic criteria for the diagnosis of depression. Thus, it seems that with the group of conjugally bereaved there is a pathologically grieving subgroup. We will not speculate in this paper on the reasons for a pathological outcome following the death of a spouse. Deutsch (1937), Karasu and Waltzmann (1976), and Kübler-Ross (1973) have all addressed themselves to that issue. They caution that any intervention in the grieving process should be carefully considered, because it may cause an inhibition of the grief, leading to a pathological grief reaction. This caution is both an observation on the mourning process and a warning to physicians who might be inclined to intervene, especially with medications. Is such advice sound?

It is our contention that normal grief is a severe disappointment reaction and that at least one form of pathological grief is a precipitated endogenomorphic depression. According to the conceptualization of Klein (1974), disappointment reaction is a phasic dysphoric reaction clearly in response to a stress, such as frustration or loss. The reaction is usually self-limited, and although there may be a persistent dysphoric mood, vegetative symptoms are mainly absent.

Klein's *endogenomorphic depression* is analogous to the commonly used term *endogenous depression* in that the core psychopathological elements are a persistent loss of ability to enjoy usually pleasant activities and a loss of interest in pursuing such activities. Physiological behavioral concomitants are common: the "vegetative" symptoms of insomnia, weight loss, dry mouth, agitation or retardation, easy fatigability, diminished ability to concentrate, and diurnal variation. The difference from the usual conception of endogenous depression is that the term endogenomorphic is meant to imply that the presence or absence of a precipitant is not relevant, that the association of "endogenous" features with the absence of a precipitant is a misleading association. The value of Klein's conceptualization is that it explains better the drug research data, in which the presence or absence of a precipitant does not predict drug responsiveness, while the "endogenous" clinical features do.

If what we assert is true, that grief is a disappointment reaction and pathological mourning is endogenomorphic depression, then the relevance to drug treatment of grief is that antidepressants should not be effective in usual grief (disappointment reactions) and should be in pathological mourning. Several authors advise against intervention in grieving. Often sedation, through the use of minor tranquilizers or neuroleptics, is discouraged (Klerman 1973) because they oversedate the individual and do not allow for the necessary expression of affect and acceptance of the situation. Kübler-Ross (1973) comments that drugs should not replace human care. We believe that medication is not a substitute for the interaction between therapist and patient: it is a separate treatment. Both drug treatment and psychotherapy must establish their usefulness by empirical research, not by apodictic assertions.

Karasu and Waltzmann (1976) assert:

> Bereavement is . . . a state that must be dealt with psychosocially rather than psychopharmacologically . . . . Giving mourners hypnotics or antianxiety drugs to decrease their losses is an unfortunate practice, and one to be thoroughly condemned . . . . The antidepressants are of questionable value in the majority of uses, with their primary result being the production of anticholinergic side effects. Their use should be limited to those in whom the loss precipitated already existing endogenomorphic process but at the present time it is not known precisely what the pre-existing picture is.

They cite no research to substantiate these opinions, nor does Kübler-Ross (1973). Kline (1973), Klerman (1973), Hollister (1973), and Arkin (1973) all suggest the use of antidepressant medication if the depression is extremely severe. Arkin (1973) does note that drugs must be used with caution but not to suppress or avert grief; the aim of treatment is to "administer only those drugs and in such quantities that grief does not become excessively disorganizing and destructive to the person, and the person is permitted to experience, work through and endure bereavement." Again, none of these authors cites any empirical evidence as a basis for his or her opinions.

There are a few anecdotal reports of antidepressant or electroconvulsive treatment for pathological grief reactions. Clayton et al. (1968) cite one person, with a previous history of affective disorder, who responded to treatment with imipramine for a depressive episode during conjugal bereavement. Maddison and Raphael (1973) describe three people who became depressed concomitant with mourning and who evidenced insomnia, agitation or retardation, and weight loss. All three responded to treatment with tricyclic antidepressants and then returned to normal mourning. They note, as does Maickel (1973), that there is a dearth of studies to substantiate or refute the claims made to use or not use medication in bereavement. Myerson (1944) reviews four cases, and Lynn and Racy (1969), one case who became severely depressed following a loss. All five responded to electroconvulsive therapy (ECT) and subsequently reverted from the pathological state to one of more normal mourning. Lynn and Racy detail the history of the woman they studied. After the loss of her sister she had persistent sadness, anorexia with weight loss, insomnia, and constipation and was unable to perform her usual household chores. She developed the delusion that she had caused her sister's death. These symptoms did not respond to amitriptyline but did respond to electroconvulsive treatments. She was then able to accept her sister's death, was able to laugh, felt optimistic about the future, and made plans to return to work as a schoolteacher. It was clear, however, she was also grieving, because she cried when talking about her sister, visited her grave, and recalled memories of their life together. Several months after the ECT, she was fully able to enjoy her life but was still sad and tearful when talking about her sister. Though this is only a single case, it is suggestive that pathological grief is different from normal mourning, and it is noteworthy that the patient was able to experience pleasure in her life only after adequate treatment, while still grieving.

Our review of the literature revealed no systematic investigations of the appropriate treatment for depression during bereavement, though as noted above, several authors have expressed strong opinions against the use of any medication, including antidepressant medication, because "the impact of much medication for either psychodynamic or pharmacologic reasons is such that its effects may well be inhibition, the inhibition of the mourning process" (Maddison and Raphael 1973).

We are currently involved in research to begin to answer these questions. Our question is: How responsive to antidepressant medications are widows who are sufficiently depressed so that, aside from the precipitant of bereavement, they meet usual criteria for drug-sensitive illness? Using a community- and hospital-based referral system, we offer six weeks of counseling to recently bereaved widows. Widows are first seen, for several reasons, usually four weeks after the death. The first several weeks after the death are the times of maximal family contact, arranging the funeral, financial affairs, visiting relatives, and so on. Our psychotherapeutic intervention comes when these sources of support are waning. We follow the subjects weekly and explore with them the loss and their problems related to it. The widows are rated with the Hamilton Rating Scale for Depression (HRSD), the Clinical Global Impression (CGI), and the Self-reporting Symptom Inventory (SCL-90), (ECDEU Manual 1976). If the HSRD is greater than 18, we diagnose the widow, using the Research Diagnostic Criteria of Spitzer et al. (1977). Those women who meet the criteria for Major Affective Disorder are offered treatment with imipramine or placebo in double-blind fashion for six weeks. The maximum dose is 300 mg/day. Counseling is continued on a weekly basis. Those women who improve will be followed monthly thereafter. Those who do not, and were on placebo, will be offered open active medication. Those on imipramine who do not respond will be offered treatment with other antidepressants if it is felt they had an adequate therapeutic dosage of the imipramine. We predict there will be a drug effect.

We also have an interest in evaluating the neuroendocrine correlates of grief—for example, urine MHPG and human growth hormone response to insulin-induced hypoglycemia. (This aspect of the research was started by Dr. Edward Sachar and his group.) Such neuroendocrine measures are known to discriminate depressed subjects from normals. Finding out whether grieving widows will be more like the normals or the depressives, or whether within the widowed group there will be variation that correlates with the degree of resemblance to usual clinical depression, should help in our understanding of bereavement. Although there is some research in this area (Hofer 1972), it is still not conclusive enough to make predictions.

Some assert that interference with mourning could cause psychological damage. We question the concept that all mourning is a benign process. Clayton (1968) notes that 25 percent of her sample had some serious medical illness and 44 percent had seen a doctor within a year of their loss. In Parkes' study (1970), within a year 27 percent suffered a deterioration of their health, and no widow's health was clearly better. In a more recent review, Jacobs and Ostfeld (1977) conclude there is a "basic pattern of excess mortality in the widowed" and describe studies with a mortality seven times the expected rate among the conjugally bereaved.

There are, in summary, two reasons to study the value of antidepressants in grieving widows who meet criteria for clinical depression. The first is to alleviate suffering. We reject the assumed necessity for severe suffering in grief. Before omitting to relieve suffering, we should have excellent evidence that the overall assessment of risk supports such therapeutic passivity. Such evidence does not exist, and we believe the burden of proof lies upon those who, on the basis of anecdotal experience or therapeutic speculation, aver that such grief should be uninterrupted. Certainly, no evaluation of the risk-benefit ratio is possible until we know if severe grieving is drug-responsive.

The second reason is concern over the terrible mortality rate among widows. If it is true, as the data support so far, that the mortality rate is increased sevenfold in the widowed, we are dealing with a public health problem of enormous proportions. It is not known, of course, whether, if antidepressants are effective in severe grief, use of these would reduce the mortality. However, even the possibility of the effect must be tested.

References

Arkin, A. M. 1973. "The Use of Medications in the Management of the Dying Patient and in the Bereaved." In I. K. Goldberg et al., eds. (1973):72–76.
Bornstein, P. E., P. J. Clayton, J. D. Halikas, et al. 1973. "The Depression of Widowhood After Thirteen Months." *British Journal of Psychiatry* 122:561–66.
Burgess, W. A. 1976. *Community Mental Health: Target Populations.* Englewood Cliffs, N. J.: Prentice-Hall.
Clayton, P. J. 1978. Presentation at the meeting of the American Psychopathological Association, Boston (March).
Clayton, P. J., L. Desmarais, and G. Winokur. 1968. "A Study of Normal Bereavement." *American Journal of Psychiatry* 125:64–74.
Clayton, P. J., J. A. Halikas, and W., L. Maurice. 1972. "The Depression of Widowhood." *British Journal of Psychiatry* 120:71–77.
Deutsch, H. 1937. "Absence of Grief." *Psychoanalytic Quarterly* 6:12–25.
Feighner, J. P., E. Robins, S. B. Guze, et al. 1972. "Diagnostic Criteria for Use in Psychiatric Research." *Archives of General Psychiatry* 26:57–65.
Freud, S. 1957 (1917). *Mourning and Melancholia.* In *The Complete Psychological Works of Sigmund Freud,* vol. 14, London: Hogarth.
Goldberg, I. K., S. Malitz, and A. H. Kutscher, eds. 1973. *Psychopharmacologic Agents for the Terminally Ill and Bereaved.* New York: Columbia University Press.
Greenblatt, M. 1978. "The Grieving Spouse." *American Journal of Psychiatry* 135:43–58.
Hofer, M. A., C. T. Wolff, S. B. Friedman, et al. 1972. "A Psychoendocrine Study of Bereavement." *Psychosomatic Medicine* 38:481–504.
Hollister, L. E. 1973. "Psychotherapeutic Drugs in the Dying and Bereaved." In I. K. Goldberg et al., eds. (1973):65–67.
Jacobs, S. and A. Ostfeld. 1977. "An Epidemiological Review of the Mortality of Bereavement." *Psychosomatic Medicine* 39:344–57.
Karasu, T. B. and S. Waltzmann. 1976. "Death and Dying in the Aged." In L. Bellak and T. B. Karasu, eds. *Geriatric Psychiatry* New York: Grune and Stratton.
Klein, D. F. 1974. "Endogenomorphic Depression." *Archives of General Psychiatry* 31:447–54.
Klerman, G. 1973. "Drugs and the Dying Patient." In I. K. Goldberg et al., eds. (1973):14–27.
Kline, N. S. 1973. "Indications for Psychopharmacologic Management of the Dying Patient." In I. K. Goldberg et al., eds. (1973):28–31.

Kübler-Ross, E. 1973. "On the Case for Psychopharmacologic Agents for the Dying Patient and the Bereaved." In I. K. Goldberg et al., eds. (1973):3–6.
Lindemann, E. 1944. "Symptomatology and Management of Acute Grief." *American Journal of Psychiatry* 101:141–48.
Lynn, E. J. and J. Racy. 1969. "The Resolution of Pathological Grief After Electroconvulsive Therapy." *Journal of Nervous and Mental Diseases* 148:165–69.
Maddison, D. and B. Raphael. 1973. "Normal Bereavement as an Illness Requiring Care: Psychopharmacological Approaches." In I. K. Goldberg et al., eds. (1973):235–48.
Maickel, R. P. 1973. "Current Chemotherapeutic Trends and the Need for Additional Research (for the Dying and the Bereaved)." In I. K. Goldberg et al., eds. (1973):307–10.
Myerson, A. 1944. "Prolonged Cases of Grief Reaction Treated by Electric Shock." *New England Journal of Medicine* 230:255–56.
Parkes, C. M. 1970. "The First Year of Bereavement." *Psychiatry* 33:444–67.
Spitzer, R. L., J. Endicott, and E. Robins. 1977. "Research Diagnostic Criteria for a Selected Group of Functional Disorders. New York: New York State Psychiatric Institute.
U. S. Department of Health, Education, and Welfare, National Institute of Mental Health. 1976. *ECDEU Assessment Manual for Psychopharmacology,* pp. 179–92, 217–22, 333–39.
Wahl, C. W. 1970. "The Differential Diagnosis of Normal and Neurotic Grief Following Bereavement." *Psychosomatics* 11:104–6.

23.
THE RELEVANCE OF PSYCHOPHARMACOLOGIC AGENTS FOR THE BEREAVED IN A COMMUNITY MENTAL HEALTH CENTER (CMHC)

Arleen I. Skversky, Richard F. Tislow, and Anthony F. Santore

In this paper, we focus on the use of psychopharmacologic agents with patients experiencing separation and loss, as well as bereavement, and examine the role a community mental health center (CMHC) plays in the treatment process. We believe that psychopharmacologic agents are not a substitute for human care. Of primary importance is the clinical and psychosocial care of patients, psychopharmacologic agents being used only as adjunctive therapy. How our society deals with loss and grief and the way in which these cultural values have accelerated the role played by CMHCs are demonstrated in the presentation of two case histories:

Case 1
  Ms. A, who had recently lost her husband to cancer, was referred to the mental health clinic by her internist. This 59-year-old widow had suffered with several physical ailments and had been under constant care of the internist most of her life. The patient was referred for individual psychotherapy and chemotherapy. Her complaints at this time were depression, anxiety, difficulty in making decisions, sleep disturbances, and extreme sensitivity, particularly regarding the death of her husband.

Ms. A stayed in treatment with the clinic's therapist for 15 months and was seen for one hour every two weeks. During this period, she expressed concern about her inability to process the claims for financial benefits that she was entitled to. She became increasingly depressed and had severe headaches. She suffered yet another loss with the deterioration of her eyesight. Although on prescribed antidepressant and sleep medications, her symptoms were only partially reduced. Psychotherapy terminated when the therapist was transferred to another unit, and it was recommended that the patient continue with a new therapist. After several months absence from the clinic, she returned to be seen by the new therapist. During the interval, Ms. A had experienced a visual hallucination in which she saw her dead husband. She became increasingly anxious and depressed, and the medications did not appear to be helpful.

When therapy was renewed, Ms. A was most concerned with her inability to receive medical assistance and the new glasses she needed. A four-week contract was drawn between therapist and patient, and it was agreed that they would work on the management of practical problems. At the end of the four-week period, they would determine whether Ms. A needed help with other issues.

The therapist was able to resolve Ms. A's management problems in the first few sessions, which pleased the patient. In the course of these sessions, she began to reveal experiences and feelings from the past. As a child she almost died of diphtheria and was not allowed to be as active as the other children. Although angered by this, she never expressed her angry feelings, because she had been taught at home to hold in anger and turn the other cheek.

At the end of the four-week period, Ms. A requested the opportunity to work on resolving some of her feelings of loss. She seemed to be plagued not only by memories of her husband's death but also by the deaths of her mother (when she was age 16), father (age 23), a niece, and her in-laws.

Ms. A continued to see her therapist for an hour each week for the next two months. At one session she reported that a sister-in-law had robbed her of some personal belongings, and despite the fact that she was angry she felt that she should be understanding and forgiving. The therapist pointed out how typical this was of her reactions: to lose something (a mother and a husband, as well as her eyesight) and feel angry but not entitled to express anger openly. Through treatment Ms. A expressed feelings of fright and guilt related to her husband's death. The therapist was able, through a reality-testing process, to explore and test the assumptions underlying these feelings, and as a result of this approach Ms. A experienced great relief.

Around this time Ms. A began to report better sleep and less difficulty in breathing and appeared generally less anxious and depressed. By the end of the third month of treatment Ms. A discussed termination. She felt she had resolved many of her practical problems, and she now had a way of dealing with her overwhelming fears and feelings of guilt. On her own, she was now able to trace her thought processes and test her assumptions as they related to her day-to-day existence, as well as to the death of her husband.

At the end of therapy the therapist found Ms. A less anxious, less guiltridden, and able to analyze her own fears in future stressful situations.

Comment

There are several interesting points to be made in this case. First, the differing techniques and values of the therapists had an important effect on this patient. The first therapist emphasized a here-and-now approach and encouraged the patient to ventilate her feelings. On the other hand, the second therapist, who also focused on a reality-oriented approach, provided some insights and awareness to the patient's emotions and her ability to make changes in her life. The second therapist's confidence in the ability of an older adult to change was certainly of crucial importance. Secondly, the medications only partially reduced the patient's symptoms. The patient reported a significant change at the point of termination with the second therapist.

Case 2
Ms. C, a 24-year-old single mother of one child, referred herself for treatment. Her complaints were depression, lack of energy, and poor sleep. During her initial interview with the therapist the patient was slightly withdrawn but managed to talk about her preoccupation with nightmares and her concern about a baby she had lost in her eighth month of pregnancy, nine months earlier. The patient had fears about conceiving again, since the baby she lost was malformed. Ms. C told the therapist that she still sees the father of the dead infant and that they have plans to marry. To clarify the circumstances around the miscarriage, the therapist saw Ms. C in another individual session. Ms. C reported that she had never been given any explanation for why the baby was malformed and had died. During this session the possibility of genetic counseling was presented. Ms. C agreed to a referral to a genetic-counseling clinic and agreed also to

see the therapist once a week in a women's group. She was also referred and evaluated for chemotherapy.

Ms. C attended chemotherapy clinic only four times at two- and three-week intervals. Initially, she was given Sinequan 100 mg t.h.s. Later, she complained of lack of energy and poor sleep, and her medication was changed to Elavil 25 mg t.h.s. and Tofranil 25 mg in the morning and at noon. The medications partially relieved her symptoms. After being in treatment for three months, Ms. C terminated chemotherapy on her own but continued her group sessions. She felt that the medicines had helped with sleep, given her a little more energy, and eased her depression, but that now she could manage on her own.

She attended group sessions for a total of seven months. She had an opportunity to discuss the loss of her dead fetus and the horror of not understanding what happened. She related to the group that because the fetus was malformed, it was not considered a whole child and was given a funeral or memorial service. This seemed to bother her quite a bit. After five months the therapist noted that Ms. C appeared less depressed and withdrawn and was more spontaneous in group sessions. Ms. C began to talk about finding a job as a nurse's aide. Within a month she did secure such employment in a home for retarded children. She was happy with her employment and continued to function well. Two months after she secured this position, she terminated her group sessions on her own. At the point of termination she still had not gone for genetic counseling, because of a waiting list of several months. Although she was unable to be seen immediately, she did plan to pursue the referral.

Comment

Because of the inadequate explanation of the death of a malformed fetus and the lack of an opportunity to grieve for her loss, this 24-year-old woman within nine months became increasingly withdrawn and depressed. Medications partially helped at the onset of treatment with sleep and depression. But of crucial importance was the patient's opportunity, with the therapist's encouragement, to express her feelings of loss and her eventual acceptance of this loss.

Discussion

As suggested by Hollister, (1973), "the final resolution of loss by the bereaved is better accompanied by psychological help than by the use of drugs." It is human contact and care that are so crucial in helping the bereaved. Our societal values do not always encourage the individual to engage in the expression of emotional feelings and to mourn for loved ones at the time of loss. Those who are not able to grieve often experience depression and a variety of other symptoms. The role of the local community mental health center has been to provide the human contact and encouragement that help depressed people to mourn and accept their loss with understanding rather than with guilt and shame.

References

Hollister, L. E. 1973. "Psychotherapeutic Drugs in the Dying and Bereaved." In I. K. Goldberg, S. Malitz, and A. H. Kutscher, eds. *Psychopharmacologic Agents for the Terminally Ill and Bereaved.* New York: Columbia University Press, 1973. 65–71.

Index

Abel, S., 142–43
Acceptance, 182
Acetaminophen, 117
Acetyl donor, 47
ACTH, 170, 172
Acupuncture, 67
Acute pain, 19–20, 24, 71–74, 81
Addiction, 122–24; defined, 100; and drug ingestion suicide, 56–57, 58, 62; fears of, 35, 79, 81, 162, 188; irrelevant in terminal care, 149–50. *See also* Drug dependence
Addiction potential, 143, 162; of diamorphine, 75, 76, 79
Addiction Research Center (Lexington), 123
Addiction Research Center Inventory, 144
Adjustment disorder(s), 194
Adrenal steroids, 172
Adrenergic neuron blocking agents, 42
Age: and response to potent narcotics, 138
Aitken-Swan, J., 71
Akathisia, 156
Albany Medical College, 152
Albumin, 44, 45–46
Alcohol, 18, 43, 55–56, 60, 68, 128, 200
Alcoholism, 56; in bereaved, 188, 194
Alert analgesia, 148, 150
Alertness, 75, 100, 102, 144, 146, 150, 182
Alexander, I. E., 4
Alkalizing agents, 43–44
Alpha/adrenergic nervous system, 143
Alpha-adrenergic stimulants, 143
Alpha globulins, 44
American Society for Clinical Pharmacology and Therapeutics, 129
American Society of Clinical Onocology, 22
Amino acids, 25, 47
Amitriptyline, 421, 205
Amphetamine(s), 20–21, 49, 129, 136, 137, 139; analgesic properties of, 138–139; combined with opiates, 142–46. *See also* Methadone-amphetamine
Amygdala, 170
Analeptic drugs, 54
Analgesia, 38, 67, 102, 105–27; demand, 148–50; ensuring adequate, 68–69; stimulant drugs combined with opiates in, 142–47; in terminally ill, 169
Analgesic efficacy, 139; Brompton's Cocktail, 133–36
Analgesic League Table, 102
Analgesic measures: in treatment of terminal cancer, 77
Analgesics, 11, 34, 35, 55, 68, 74–75; combination, 128–41; cumulative effects of, 40; nonnarcotic, 102, 115; pharmacokinetic aspects of, in palliative care, 148–50; in relief for dying and bereaved, 151–58, 185–86; in treatment of terminal cancer, 102–3, 111–14; used on cancer ward, 160–62. *See also* Narcotic analgesics
Anderson, C., 194
Anergic depression, 194
Anesthesia, 30
Anesthetist, 67
Androgens, 110–11
Anger, 36, 73–74, 166, 168, 203; in bereavement, 182, 192

Anileridine, 101, 145–46
Animal studies, 80, 123, 143, 145, 170, 171, 172
Anorexia, 20, 75, 182, 201, 205
Antacids, 42
Antianxiety medications, 191, 195
Antibiotics, 130
Anticholinergic agents, 42
Anticipatory pain, 149, 150
Anticonvulsants, 47
Antidepressants, 54, 82, 85, 111–13, 162, 192, 195; for dying and bereaved, 154, 155, 156, 178, 185–86. *See also* Tricyclic antidepressants
Antiemetics, 52, 121; prophylactic, 111
Antihistamines, 47, 60
Antiinflammatory drugs, 114–17
Anti-Parkinson agents, 54
Antipsychotic drugs, 192
Antitussive agents, 75
Anxiety, 10, 11, 20, 108, 111, 125, 154, 182; effect on experience of pain, 65; in mourning, 190–92, 195, 201; nondrug relief for, 162–63; pretest, 161; relief of, 25, 75, 164
Anxiety-depression (coexistent), 190, 191–92, 194, 195
Anxiolytic agents, 12
Appetite, 20, 75, 115, 135–36, 138, 200
Arkin, A. M., 187, 193, 204–5
Aspirin, 43–44, 55, 68, 74, 80, 160; and opium, 118; in relief of bone pain, 114–17
Aspirin-codeine, 118
Assessment of pain, 106–10, 125, 126
Ataxia, 42
Attitudinal change: in treatment of dying, 4
Autopsy, 26, 56

Balter, M. B., 151
Barbiturates, 36, 47, 178, 190; in drug overdose, 53, 54–55, 56, 60
Basal ganglia function, 170
Beaver, W. T., 80
Becker, E., 4
Bedsores, 108
Beecher, H. K., 35, 36, 65, 101
Behavioral modification, 18

Belief systems: in healing, 31–32; of medical staff, 21–22, 31–32. *See also* Value systems
Bellville, J. W., 138
Benzodiazepine hypnotics, 193
Benzodiazepine tranquilizers, 178
Benzodiazepines, 60, 190, 192
Bereaved (the), 9, 34, 36–37; identification of high-risk, 179–81, 183; psychopharmacologic agents and analgesics in relief for, 151–58; psychotropic medication for, 10, 12, 187, 188
Bereavement: potential pathogenic effect of, 179; psychiatric complications in, 194–96; psychopharmacologic treatment of, 185–99; tricyclic antidepressants in treatment of depression in, 200–8
Beta-endorphin, 170–71, 172
Beta globulins, 44
Bile, 50
Biogenic amines, 143
Biological school of thought, 3
Birtchnell, J., 179
Birth, 172, 173
Bivalent cations, 44
Bond, M. R., 68
Bone marrow depression, 160
Bone pain, 110–11, 114–17, 126
Bornstein, P. E., 202
Bowen, A., 186
Brain: in near-death experience, 169–74
Brain stem, 170
Breast cancer, 110, 125
Breathlessness, 182
British Medical Journal, 73, 128
British National Formulary, 119
Brompton's Cocktail(s), 108–19, 128, 129–40
Brompton's Hospital, 128
Brompton's Mixture, 161
Bronchial carcinoma, 125
Brown, R. J., 186, 188, 194
Bunch, J., 194
Bunyard, P., 99
Burgess, W. A., 203
Burn, J. I., 103
Butyrophenone, 66

Index

Caffeine, 43
Calvinism, 13
Cancer, 20, 38; pain control in treatment of, 65–69, 128–41
Cancer, terminal: narcotic analgesics in treatment of, 79–104; diamorphine in management of, 70–127
Cancer patients, 24; limitations of psychotropic drugs in treatment of, 28–33
Cancer ward, 159–63
Carcinoma: of breast, bronchus, prostate, 110
Carcinomata: of kidney, thyroid, 110
Cardiorespiratory arrest: resuscitation from, 169
Cardiotoxicity, 55
Cardiovascular toxicity, 138
Care: in bereavement, 178, 187, 204; concept of, in hospitals, 163; in loss, separation, 210, 213–214
Caring, 26; in suicide prevention, 61
Carr, D., 172
Cathartics, 42
Central nervous system, (CNS) 17–18, 25, 143; subsystems, 7–8; neurotransmitter concentrations, 139
Central nervous system (CNS) stimulants, 129, 137, 138, 139, 140
Cerebellar subsystem, 7
Cerebral cortex, 170
Chelating agents, 44
Chemical neurolysis, 124
Chemotherapy, 21, 29, 110, 159, 160
Chlordiazepoxide, 54, 55–56, 190
Chlorpromazine, 8, 66, 74, 82, 102, 119, 161, 192
Chlortetracycline, 50
Cholestyramine, 44
Chronic pain, 20, 65, 71–74, 81, 102
Chronically ill (the): demand analgesia for, 149
Cinchona bark, 35
Clayton, P. J., 188, 190, 193, 194, 201–2, 205, 207
Clergy, 11, 152–58
Clift, A. D., 193
Clinical Global Impression (CGI), 206
Clinical pharmacology, 22

Clinical tests: needed, in use of diamorphine, 103; of stimulant drugs combined with opiatess, 142–43
Clorazepate, 190
Cocaine, 74, 82, 103, 118–19, 129, 140, 146; and opium, 128; oral absorption of, 137. *See also* Methadone-cocaine
Cocaine pharmacokinetics, 137
Codeine, 80, 115, 118, 160–61
Cognitive confusion, 11, 12
Cognitive structures, 7
Comfort, 15
Communication, 15; use of medications and, 166–68
Companionship, 113
Conjugal bereavement, 200–8
Constant-infusion pumps, 149
Constipation, 108, 121, 135, 182, 205
Continuing care: diamorphine in, 105–27
Controlled substances, 151–52
Coping ability, 30
Cortical neuro-psychological subsystems, 7
Corticosteroids, 115
Cortisone, 166
Cosynthesized peptides, 172
Cough, 82
Coumarin anticoagulants, 45
Cousins, N., 28
Counseling: for widow, 206
Covi, L., 192
Cox, P. R., 194
Crawford, M. E., 69
Crisis intervention, 61, 62
Crisp, A. H., 190
Crying, 201
Cultural differences, 10
Cumulative Index Medicus, 185
Cyclizine, 118, 121
Cystitis, 108
Cytochrome P-450, 47
Cytotoxic agents, 102, 123

Dalmane, 160, 193
Davis, J., 54
Death, 3–4, 5, 182; attitudes toward, 3–4, 11; natural, 156; premature, through pharmacology, 19–20, 146;

Death (*Continued*), reality of, 30, 35
Delta-9-tetrahydrocannabinol (THC), 22, 3, 25
Demerol, 25, 160, 162
Deneau, G., 143
Denial: in bereaved, 182; of death, 10, 11; by medical staff, 35, 167; of pain, 11, 12
Dependency, 9, 149, 150; on medication, 11–12
Depersonalization, 4, 72
Depression, 10, 11, 20, 111–13, 125, 146, 154, 164; in bereavement, 182, 200–8; in drug addiction, 57; in dying patients, 15; intensifies experience of pain, 65, 66–67; in mourning, 190, 191–92, 194–95, 214; and prescription of medication in suicide prevention, 59; tricyclic antidepressants in treatment of, in conjugal bereavement, 200–8
Despair, 20, 203
Despondency, 20, 25
Detachment, 15
Detachment from reality, 99, 100
Detoxification, 46
Deutsch, H., 186–87, 203
Dexamethasone, 115
Dexedrine, 21
Dextroamphetamine, 67, 142, 143, 144–45
Dextromoramide, 118
Dextropropoxyphene, 74
Diacetyl morphine, 118
Dialysis, 53, 54, 55
Diamorphine: dose, 82–98, 100, 101–2, 120T, 123, 24; by injection, 74, 82, 83, 98–99, 102, 119; in management of terminal cancer, 70–127; oral administration, 74, 77, 82, 83, 98, 101, 118–119; problems in use of, 75–78; in treatment of cancer pain, 118–27
Diazepam, 108, 190
Diconal, 118
Diethyl morphine, 129
Diflunisal, 115
Digitalis, 35
Digoxin, 50, 51

Dihydrocodeine, 115, 118
Dilaudid, 132–33, 160
DiMascio, A., 192
Diphenylhydantoin, 12
Dipipanone, 118
Dirksen, R. M., 172
Disappointment reaction: grief as, 203, 204
Disease, 29; multiple, 38; reality of, 32
Disruption, 30, 31, 32
Diuretics, 38–39
Diversional activity (therapy), 77, 102, 121–22
Dole, V. P., 69
Donlon, P. T., 55
Dopamine, 139
Dorpat, T L., 56
Dorsal horn, 18
Dose (dosage), 11, 12, 115; bound-to-free ratio and, 45–46; Brompton's Cocktails study, 129, 133, 135, 136, 138, 140; diamorphine, 82–98, 100, 101–2, 120T, 123–24; drugs in treatment of mourning, 191; effective, 74, 113–14; escalation of, 75–77, 79, 81; morphine, 119, 120T; radiation therapy, 111
Dosing cycle, 149
Double-blind trials, 67, 75, 130, 143–44, 145, 206
Droperidol, 66
Drug absorption: factors affecting, 42–44, 51–52
Drug abuse, 151, 157
Drug automatism, 56, 62
Drug combinations, 115, 118–19; stimulant drugs with opiates, 142–47; in treatment of bereavement, 195
Drug dependence, 151–52; defined, 100, 122; with diamorphine, 100–1
Drug distribution: factors affecting, 42, 44–46, 51–52
Drug excretion, 44, 46; factors affecting, 42, 48–50, 52
Drug interactions, 38–40, 42, 47, 54, 55–56, 60, 195; in pain relief, 66, 67, 80; prediction of adverse, 50–52
Drug metabolism, 44; factors affecting, 42, 46–48, 51–52

Drug overdose: suicide by, 53–62
Drug reactions (adverse), 39, 41–42
Drug solubility, 43–44
Drug therapy: psychological hazards of, 34–37
Drugs, 30–31, 35, 42; common in overdose, 53–56; concerns of physicians and patients with, 38–40; experimental use of, 25; nonnarcotic, 25; pain-relieving, 65–69; review of, 21–24; in treatment of grief, 200–8; *See also* Polypharmacy
Dundee, J. W., 66
Duromorph, 119
Dying (process), 151
Dying (the), 34–37; meaning of death to, 11; needs of, 15–18; psychological response in, 169–74; psychopharmacologic agents and analgesics in relief for, 151–58; psychopharmacologic treatment of, in General Systems Theory, 3–14
Dysphoria, 75
Dyspnea, 82, 99
Dystonic, 156

Ectopic parathyroid hormone, 114
Eddy, N. B., 101
Egalitarianism, 4
Egbert, L. D., 36
Ego-identity, 8
Eissler, K. R., 4
Elderly (patients), 119, 121. 192; drug problems in treatment of, 39–40
Electroconvulsive (ECT) therapy, 205
Emergency room personnel, 61
Emotional reaction to pain, 111–13
Endogenomorphic depression, 203–4
Endogenous depression: in bereavement, 192, 194, 195
Endogenous opioids, 139
England: heroin use in, 23–24
Enkephalin kinetics, 139
Environment: and analgesic response, 139
Epinephrine, 53
Epstein, G., 188
Erikson, E. H., 8
Estrogens, 110–11

Ethereal sulfates, 47
Ethnic background: and pain control, 67
Euphoria, 75, 144–45, 146, 169
Euphoriant drugs, 111
Euthanasia, 25
Evans, W. O., 143
Existentialism, 4
Exogenous depression, 195, 203–4
Expectations (patients): as to relief of pain, 125–26
Expired air, 50
Extended family system, 6, 7
Extrapyramidal motoric system, 7

Faden, A. I., 172
Familial system, 6, 7, 8
Family(ies), 3, 4, 5, 182; General Systems Theory, in treatment of, 9–13; postbereavement support service for 179–81; and suicide prevention, 60–61
Family/general practice, 58–59
Family physician, 11, 157
Farberow, N. L., 4
Fatigue, 200
FDA Drug Bulletin, 58
Fear(s), 10, 108; of death, 111, 182; of dying, 111, 182; in loss, 212; in mourning, 190; of pain, 113
Feifel, H., 4
Feighner, J. P., 202
Fentanyl, 66
Ferguson, T., 186, 189, 190
Ferreira, S. H., 114
Fever, 172
Field dependence/independence, 67–68
First-pass effect, 48
Flach, E., 32
Fluphenazine, 8
Flurazepam (Dalmane), 160, 193
Flurbiprofen, 115
Flynn, P., 32
Follow-up care: for attempted suicides, 61
Food and Drug Administration (FDA), 20, 21–22, 23
Ford, J. R., 194
Forrest, W. H., 67, 129, 144, 145

Frantz, A. G., 171
Fraser, H. F., 100
Frederick, C., 57
Free will, 8-9, 13
Freud, S., 3, 186, 200
Frontal-prefrontal organized motor conceptual structures, 7
Frosch, W. A., 57
Frustration, 62, 203
Function (system), 6, 7

Gahwiler, B. H., 171
Galasko, C. S. B., 103
Gann, D. S., 171
Gardos, G., 192
Gate control theory of pain, 139
General Systems Theory, 5-9; and psychopharmacologic treatment of dying patient, 3-14
Gentamicin, 51
Glucocorticosteroids, 84
Glucuronic acid, 47
Glutethimide, 54
Goldberg, I. K., 178, 186
Goldberg, M. R., 185
Goodman, L. S., 142, 145
Gramlich, E., 185
Greenberg, I. M., 4, 5
Greenblatt, M., 203
Greyson, B., 169, 170, 172
Grief, 151, 186-87; acute, 177-84; delayed, 187; inhibition of, 201, 203; management of, 185; normal/pathological, 200-8; suppression of, 187, 205; working through of, 36
Grief reaction, pathological, 203
Grieving, *See* Mourning
Grof, S., 24
Grosser, G. H., 187
Grotjahn, M., 4
Group for the Advancement of Psychiatry (GAP), 4, 12
Group therapy, 167-68, 210-14
Guanethidine, 42
Guilt feelings, 212

Habituation to narcotic action: metabolic rather than pharmacological, 149-50

Hall, R. C., 192
Hallucinations, 135, 138, 170, 202
Haloperidol, 24
Hamilton, A., 172
Hamilton Rating Scale for Depression, (HRSD), 206
Hanks, G. W., 66
Haroldsson, E., 169, 170, 172
Harris, S. C., 143
Harvard Bereavement Study, 179, 180
Hazinski, T. A., 172
Head cancers, 115
Headache, 115, 200
Healing, 29, 31
Health, 29, 31
Hemorrhage, 172
Henderson-Hasselbalch equations, 43
Henriksen, S., 170, 171
Henry, B. W., 192
Hepatocyte, 46, 47
Herman, S., 149
Heroin, 23-24, 118, 128, 146
Herring, P. C., 170
Hiccoughs, 161
Hippocampal seizures, 170, 171
Hippocampus, 170
Hippocrates, 35
Hofer, M. A., 207
Holaday, J. W., 172
Holistic treatment, 32, 34
Hollister, L. E., 192, 193, 204, 213
Home-centered terminal care, 105-6
Hopelessness, 57, 58, 203
Hormone treatment, 110-11
Hospice movement, 35, 128
Hospital-centered terminal care, 105-6
Hostility: treatment of, 192
Houde, R., 146
Hughes, J. C., 171
Human needs, 4, 34
Human studies: narcotic analgesics, 123; stimulants combined with opiates, 143-46
Hunt, J. M., 125, 126
Hypercalcemia, 103, 114
Hypertension, 42
Hypnosis, 12, 67, 68, 148
Hypnotic agents, nonbarbiturate, 53, 54-55, 60; prescriptions for, 58, 59

Hypnotics, 67, 193
Hypoalbuminemia, 46, 51
Hypoglycemia, 207
Hypotension, 172
Hypothalamus, 7, 170

Illich, Ivan: *Medical Nemesis*, 30
Illness: attitudes toward, 8
Imipramine, 42, 66–67, 205, 206
Immobilization, 110, 124–25
Impotence, 29, 31, 32
Indomethacin, 117
Informed consent, 21
Inhabituation, 193
Inhalation anesthesia, 24–25
Injections, 161. *See also* Diamorphine, by Injection
Insensitivity, 34
Insomnia, 190, 200, 205
Intactness (system), 6
Integrative structures, 7
Intensity of pain, 108–10, 149, 150
Interactional processes (systems), 7
Internal fixation, 125
Internal medicine, 58–59
Interpersonal field system, 6
Interpersonal interaction system, 8
Intrapsychic beliefs, 12, 14
Intrapsychic system, 8
Isbell, H., 123
Isonipecaine, 142
Ivy, A. C., 142

Jacobs, S., 207
Jaffe, J. R., 192
Jasinski, D. R., 144
Johns, M. W., 193

Kalish, R. A., 185
Karasu, T. B., 203, 204
Keeri-Szanto, M., 149
Kellner, R., 190, 191, 192, 195
Kidney, 49, 50
Klein, D. F., 203, 204
Klerman, G., 204
Kline, N. S., 204
Krant, M. J., 188
Kraus, A. S., 194
Krieger, D. T., 170–71

Kübler-Ross, E., 4, 178, 187, 189, 203, 204
Kuhar, M. J., 171
Kutscher, A. H., 185
Kutscher, L. G., 185

Laetrile, 168
Lamerton, R., 182
Lasagna, L., 101, 140
Lavage, 53
Laycock, J. D., 71
Lee, L. E., 101
Lehmann, H. E., 145
Lennard, H. L., 151
LeShan, L., 72
Levarterenol, 53
Levorphanol, 119–21, 124
Lewis, J. W., 170
Lidocaine, 48
Life after life, 169
Life support, 25–26
Lifestyle: modification of, 124–25
Lilienfeld, A. M., 194
Limbic lobe syndrome, 170–73
Limbic system, 7, 8, 170
Lime juice, 35
Lindemann, E., 187, 192, 194, 201, 203
Liver, 46, 48
Liver disease, 51
Living will, 25
Lorr, M., 190
Loss, 13, 189, 203, 210–14
LSD, 24, 57, 67, 148
Luria, A. R., 7
Lutkins, S. G., 36, 194
Lynn, E. J., 205

McCourt, W. E., 185
MacMahon, B., 194
McNair, D. M., 190
Maddison, D., 185, 187, 189, 205, 206
Maickel, R. P., 205
Malaise, 11
Malignant melanoma, 125
Manic depressives, 20
Mania, 194
Marijuana, 151–52
Marris, P., 190, 192, 193
Martin, J. B., 170

Martindale, 128
Massive hepatic metastases, 115
Meaninglessness: of/in chronic pain, 72, 81
Medical Nemesis (Illich), 30
Medical staff: as advocates for patients, 26; attitude toward dying patient, 10–11; dealing with feelings in face of death 37; patients' pain transmitted to, 19, 31, 34–35, support by, 18, 29–30. *See also* Nurses; Physician(s)
Medication(s), 11, 12, 36; adjuvant, 102, 121–22; belief systems and, 13, 21–22; denial of need for, 8; escalation of, 140 (*see also* Dose [dosage]); frequent and regular administration of, 35, 68–69, 81, 82, 102, 113; oral, pharmacology of, 51, 102, 161; purpose of, 164; resistance to use of, 13; as substitute for physician/patient relationship, 36, 37, 204; tailored to individual, 157; used on cancer ward, 160–63; *See also* Drugs; Overmedication; Undermedication
Melancholia, 200
Melzack, R., 139
Mental faculties: impairment of, from narcotic analgesics, 81, 99–100. *See also* Alertness
Mental health workers, 152–58
Mental suffering: in chronic pain, 72–74, 75
Meperidine, 142, 145
Meprobamate, 54
Merlis, S., 195
Merritt, H. H., 170
Mesoridazine, 55
Metabolites, 46, 48, 49, 114
Methadone, 57, 69, 121, 123, 128–41, 161–62; as analgesic, 140
Methadone-amphetamine, 128–41
Methadone-cocaine, 128–41
Methotrimeprazine: intramuscular, 140
Metoclopramide, 121
Microinfusion pump(s), 69
Microsomal enzymes, 46–47
Midbrain, 170
Middlesex Health Questionnaire, 190
Milton, G. W., 100

Modification of pathological process, 110–11
Moertal, C. G., 80
Molecular oxygen, 46–47
Monoamine oxides (MAO) inhibitors, 20, 54, 67, 195
Mood, 75, 117, 171
Moody, R. A., 169, 170, 172
Moore, J., 66
Morbidity, risk of, 41; in bereaved, 36
Morphine, 17, 25, 35–36, 66, 80, 102, 108, 114, 118, 160, 162; administration by continuous extradural infusion, 69; in combination with other drugs (pain relief), 66, 67; combined with amphetamine, 142, 143–45; criterion for prescription of, 114; fear of addiction to, 122–23; optimal dose, 101; oral administration, 118, 119; oral dose, 113–14; subcutaneous, 101
Mortality: in bereaved, 36, 188, 194, 207–8; as intrapsychic matter, 4
Motor cortex, 170
Mourning, 36, 200, 214; inhibition of, 206; interference with, 186–87, 207; intervention in, 203, 204; psychopharmacologic treatment of, 189–93; symptoms in, 201
Movement: and pain, 124–26
Muller, C., 151
Muller-Fahlbusch, H., 194
Multiple myeloma, 110, 114
Mundy, G. R., 114
Murphy, G. E., 59, 194
Murray, P., 31
Musculoskeletal disorders, 108
Myerson, A., 205
Myocardial infarction, 8

NADPH, 47
Nalorphine hydrochloride, 101
Naloxone hydrochloride, 55
Narcotic analgesics, 66, 115, 118–21; confusion about, 79, 80; criterion for prescription of, 114; and depression, 111; effect of stimulants on, 139; long-term effects of, 123; potentiated by CNS stimulants, 129; synthetic, 101; use and abuse of, in treatment of

terminal cancer, 79–104
Narcotic-CNS stimulant combinations, 129, 139–40
Narcotics, 11, 22–24, 25, 67; around-the-clock use of, 24; oral analgesic equivalence of, 121T; schedule of administration of, 68–69; synthetic, 74
National Health Service, 177
National Institute of Mental Health, 23
Nausea, vomiting, 16, 111, 118, 121, 135, 140, 144, 161, 182; control of, 82, 101, 133, 142; physician-patient relationship and, 15–16; from treatment, 71, 74
Near-death experience, 169–74
Neck cancers, 117
Negative thinking, 182
Neonates, 50, 143
Nepenthe, 118
Nerve blocks, 102, 123, 124, 148
Nerve compression, 115, 124
Neuroendocrine correlates of grief, 207
Neurolepanalgesia (NLA), 66
Neuroleptic (antipsychotic) drugs, 65–66, 204
Neurologic events: near-death experiences as, 169–74
Neurologists, 7
Neurology, 59
Neuropsychiatric disturbances, 115
Neuropsychiatrists, 7, 8
Neurons: pain-carrying, 17–18
Neurosurgeon(s): on pain control team, 67
Neurosurgery, 77
Neurotic depression, 12
Neurotransmitters, 7, 143
Newman-Keuls Tests, 154–55
Nickerson, M., 142, 145
Nitrous oxide, 67
Nonionized lipid-soluble drug forms, 43, 44
Nonsteroidal antiinflammatory drugs (NSAID), 114, 140
Norepinephrine, 42, 139
Nuclear family system, 6, 7, 9
Nurses, 10; on cancer ward, 162–63; and suicide prevention in drug overdose, 61
Nutt, J. G., 144
Nystagmus, 42
Nyswander, M. E., 69

Obsessive ruminative thinking, 15
O'Donnell, J. A., 57
Oncology patients: limitations of psychotropic drugs in treatment of, 28–33
Opiates: stimulant drugs combined with, 142–47
Opioid peptides, 171
Opium, 35, 118, 128, 178, 185
Organism(s): as index system, 6–7
Osis, K., 169, 170, 172
Osseous metastasis, 110–11, 114–17
Osteoclast activating factor, 114
Osteolysis, 114
Osteolytic cancer, 24
Ostfeld, A., 207
Overall, J. E., 192
Overmedication, 39
Oxazepam, 190, 192
Oxycodone pectinate, 119
Oxymorphone, 101
Oyama, T., 171

Paddock, R., 80
Pain, 10, 11, 12, 38, 68; diamorphine in treatment of, 70–127; facts about, 19–20; intractable, 113; meaning of, to patient, 29–32, 65; pharmacologic treatment of, 13 (*see also* Pharmacotherapy); physiology of, 17–18, 19; prevention of, 35, 102, 113; as psychobiologic phenomenon, 81; reality of, 32, 35; response to, 29–30. *See also* Acute pain; Chronic pain
Pain behavior: factors in, 65–66
Pain chart(s), 106–7, 116–17F
Pain control, 110–25, 182; complications in success of, 164–68; practical and philosophical concepts of, 19–27; in treatment of cancer, 65–69
Pain control team(s), 67
Pain-depression-pain cycle, 66
Pain experience, 68, 139
Pain-free, 69, 74, 102, 113;

Pain-free (*Continued*), graded relief in, 125–26
Pain management, 15, 17–18: philosophy underlying pharmacologic and analgesic approach to, 28–33
Pain pathways: interruption of, 110, 124
Pain reactivity, 68
Pain relief, 38; objective of, 148
Pain research, 17–18, 32, 67–69
Pain sensitivity, 25
Pain stimulus, 65, 139
Pain threshold, 25; elevation of, 110, 111–13; factors affecting, 111, 112T; peripheral, 114
Palliative care, 148–50
Papaveretum, 118
Paracetamol, 74, 80, 115, 118
Paracetamol-propoxyphene, 118
Parkes, C. M., 105, 177, 179, 186, 187, 188, 189, 190, 192, 193, 194, 201–2, 207
Passive-dependent personality, 58
Passivity, 169
Pathological fracture, 125
Pathological grief, 200–8; features of, 203
Patient(s): attitude toward drug therapy, 156–57; in Brompton's Cocktail study, 130, 132–33, 138; concerns of, with drugs, 38–40; as participant in healing process, 29, 31, 32, 135; as participant in pain control, 17, 68, 150; problem, 148; respect for, as individual(s), 73, 182; self-assessment of pain, 68; *See also* Dying (the)
Patterson, R. D., 185
Paul, N. L., 187
Pelletier, K., 31
Pelvic malignancy, 117
Penicillin, 49
Penn, C. R. H., 111
Pentazocine, 74, 80, 81, 118
Pentazocine derivatives, 25
Peptide hormones: behaviorally active, 169–74
Peptic ulcer, 108
Perception of pain, 65, 111
Peretz, D., 192

Perkoff, G. T., 172
Personality (patient), 20
Pethidine/meperidine, 118
Petrie, A., 68
pH, 43; urine, 48, 49
Pharmacokinetic aspects of analgesis in palliative care, 148–50
Pharmacologic agents: as barriers or tools, 164–68
Pharmacologic effects of drugs: free concentrations in, 44–46
Pharmacology, 22
Pharmacotherapy, 151; in bereavement, 185, 189–93
Phasic dysphoric reaction, 203
Phenazocine, 74, 119–21, 124
Phenobarbital, 42, 47, 54
Phenobarbital toxicity, 49
Phenothiazine syrup, 74
Phenothiazine tranquilizers, 25
Phenothiazines, 24, 47, 53, 82, 84–85, 102, 133, 140
Phenylbutazone, 45, 115
Phenytoin, 42, 46
Physical dependence, 122, 123, 124; with diamorphine, 101
Physician(s), 10; advocacy, 26; attitude toward use of psychopharmacologic and analgesic agents for dying and bereaved, 152–58; balance in involvement of, 34–35; concerns of, with drugs, 38–40, 41; and dying patient, 106, 111; impact of, on pain and suffering, 35–37; interest and concern by, 15, 34–35; role of, 18, 20, 21–22, 163, 196; and suicide prevention for drug ingesters, 58–61; understanding of chronic pain, 72; view of acute grief, 177–84; and withdrawal of life support, 25–26
Physician-patient relationship, 15–17, 165–67
Physiological behavior: in grief, 203
Pierce, J. I., 57
Pilowsky, I., 68
Pituitary gland, 171–72
Placebo(s), 144, 206
Placebo effect, 21, 25, 35–36
Plasma proteins, 44–45, 46, 51

Index

Polypharmacy: problem of, 38–40, 41–52
Pontine glioma, 108–10
Postoperative pain, 17, 35, 36, 66, 80, 143–44, 145, 149
Postural hypotension, 156
Powerlessness, 29
Predestination, 11
Prednisolone, 115, 124
Prednisone, 84, 103
Pregnancy, 16
Prescriptions: and suicide prevention for drug ingesters, 58–60
Prevention of pain (prevention therapy), 35, 102, 113
Priest, R. G., 190
Pro re nata (PRN, as required) basis of treatment, 76, 81, 102, 113
Prochlorperazine, 74, 82, 102, 119, 121
Proladone suppositories, 119
Promazine, 82
Propoxyphene, 48, 80
Propoxyphene napsylate, 55
Propranalol, 48
Prostaglandins (PG), 114, 115
Prosthesis(es), 125
Protein-binding sites, 44–45, 46
Proteinuria, 46
Psychiatric complications: in bereavement, 194–96
Psychiatric decompensation, 13
Psychiatric disease, disorder, 3, 12; in bereaved, 189, 194; delayed grieving and, 187
Psychiatric intervention: for dying and bereaved, 151
Psychiatric scales, 20
Psychiatrist(s), 55, 157; on pain control team, 67; and treatment of bereaved, 186–87
Psychiatry, 59
Psychic energizers, 20, 21, 24
Psychodynamic school of thought, 3
Psychodynamics: of oral ingestion suicidal behavior, 58, 62
Psychological addiction: to diamorphine, 76, 100–1
Psychological aspects of pain, 81, 102
Psychological dependence, 122

Psychological help: in loss, 213–14
Psychological treatment of dying patient, 3, 5
Psychologists: and treatment of bereaved, 186–87
Psychology: of drug addiction, 57
Psychometric tests, 20
Psychopharmacologic agents: in relief for dying and bereaved, 151–58, 177–78, 210–14
Psychopharmacologic treatment: of bereavement, 185–999; of dying patient (in General Systems Theory), 3–14
Psychophysiologic symptoms: in mourning, 190
Psychosis, 154; bereavement and, 194–95
Psychosomatic disorders: in bereavement, 194
Psychotherapeutic intervention(s) with families, 10
Psychotherapy, 204, 210–14; in bereavement, 12, 194, 196
Psychotic episodes, 12
Psychotropic drugs, 151; in bereavement, 10, 12, 187, 188, 189, 191, 194; limitations of, in supportive treatment of oncology patients, 28–33
Psychotropic medication, 5, 10, 163; in systems theory, 7–8
Pugh, T. F., 194
Punishment for sin, 11, 13
Puritanical morality, 11, 12, 13

Quality (system), 6, 7
Quality of life, 20

Racy, J., 205
Rada, R. T., 55
Radiation, 123
Radiation therapy, 29, 110, 111, 130, 159
Radiotherapy, 102
Raphael, B., 187, 189, 205, 206
Raskin, A., 194
Reaction component (in pain), 65–66
Reactive depression, 194–95
Reassurance, 12
Recovery, 30, 32

Rees, W. D., 36, 185–86, 192, 194
Reflexes: in birth, death, 172–73
Religion, 4, 13
Renal disease, 51
Renal tubular injury, 24–25
Research Diagnostic Criteria, 206
Reserpine, 143
Resistance (to treatment), 29
Reticular system, 7, 8
Reticulosis, 114
Rickles, K., 190
Robbie, D. S., 80, 118
Robins, E., 194
Rolandic sensory-motor subsystem, 7
Rossier, J., 171
Roth, M., 190
Rush, Benjamin, 178, 185
Rushing, W. A., 194
Russell, Ritchie, 77–78
Ryan, H. F., 192

Sachar, Edward, 207
St. Christopher's Hospice (London), 71, 73, 74, 76, 81–89, 100, 106, 123, 146, 179, 180, 182
St. Joseph's Hospice (London), 71, 73, 74
Saliva, 50
Salvation, belief in, 4, 11
Samarasinghe, J., 80, 118
Sarmousakis, G., 185
Saunders, C., 35, 71, 182, 183, 185
Schizophrenia, 55, 194
Schmale, A. H., Jr., 189
Scofield, P. B., 76
"Screaming room," 178
Sedation, 18, 36, 38, 42, 82, 138, 145, 146; for bereaved, 178, 187, 201, 204
Sedative hypnotics, 58
Sedatives, 20, 40, 60; in treatment of bereaved, 188
Self-esteem, 58, 203
Self-reporting Symptom Inventory (SCL-90), 206
Sensitivity, 30
Separation: use of psychopharmacologic agents in, 210–14
Septum, 170

Sequestering agents, 44
Serenity, 15
Shader, R. I., 192
Shapiro, A. K., 35
Sheehan, D. V., 195
Shneidman, E. S., 4
Shock, 172
Showalter, C. R., 187
Side effects, 8, 21, 23, 51, 101, 110, 145; of acute pain, 20; of antidepressants, 204; of benzodiazepine, 192; of Brompton's Cocktails, 135–36, 139, 140; from drugs, 39, 42; of opiates, 142, 143; of psychopharmacologic and analgesic drugs, 156–57, 158; psychotomimetic, 118; tricyclic drugs, 192
Sin, 13
Sleep, 62, 108
Sleep disturbances, 135–36, 138, 201; in mourning, 193
Smith, R. P., 143
Snow, Herbert, 128
Social group, 6, 7
Social ideology, 5
Social setting: of pain, 18
Social suffering: with chronic pain, 72, 73, 75
Social systems, 7, 10
Societal values: loss and grief in, 210, 214
Society, 6, 210, 214
Somatic complaints, 200
Spinal cord, 170
Spitzer, R. L., 206
Spouse(s), 36, 108. *See also* Widows
Sprott, N. A., 71
Staff. *See* Medical staff
Steady-state conditions, 48, 51
Steckel, Steve, 129
Stein, Z., 179, 194
Stern, K., 192
Sterols, 114
Stevenson, I., 169, 170, 172
Stimulant drugs, 53; combined with opiates, 142–47
Stress, 171, 203; in therapeutic environment, 159
Strong Memorial Hospital (Rochester,

N. Y.), 140
Structure (system), 6, 7
Study design: Brompton's Cocktails study, 130
Subcortical structures, 7
Subsystem dysfunction, 5–9
Subsystems: human being, 6–7
Suffering, 35; with chronic pain, 72, 75; ennobling aspect of, 18; in grief, 207; as means of pain mastery and control of life, 30; value of, 11
Suicidal thoughts, 201
Suicide, 4; by drug overdose, 53–62
Suicide prevention: for drug ingesters, 58–62
Suicide rates: and bereavement, 194, 195
Sulfonylureas, 47
Supersystems, 6
Support, 113; by medical staff, 18, 29–30
Support service: postbereavement family, 179–81
Support systems: for families and friends, 166; for patients, 162–63
Suppositories, 101; morphine, 119
Surgeon(s): on pain control team, 67
Survival: programmed, 26
Susser, M., 179, 194
Symptoms: of dying patient, 11; in mourning distress, 189–90, 195
Synergism: stimulant drugs/ opiates, 143, 145
System dysfunction, 5, 8–9; critical, 5, 8, 9–10; primary, 5, 8, 9; secondary, 5, 8
Systems: interactions between, 7. *See also* General Systems Theory

Takagi, H., 143
Tardive dyskinesia, 192
Tears, 50
Technology, 31, 32
Temazepan (Restoril), 193
Temporal lobe epilepsy, 8
Temporal-parietal structures, 7
Tension, 15, 62
Terminal care: and acute grief, 181–83; diamorphine in, 105–27
Terminally ill (the): demand analgesia for, 149–50. *See also* Dying (the)

Tetrabenazine, 143
Tetracyclines, 44, 50
Theophylline, 50
Thioridazine, 8, 55, 192
Thomas splints, 125
Time relationships (systems), 6–9
Tolerance, 75–77, 81, 113, 122–23, 193; with diamorphine, 85–98, 100–1, 124; to methadone, 140
Total patient care (concept), 182
Tourniquet pain technique, 145–46
Toxicity, 46
Tractotomies, 148
Tranquilizers, 82, 111; in drug overdose, 53–54, 55; in mourning, 204; prescriptions for, and suicide prevention, 59, 60; as substitute for physician's involvement, 34–35; in treatment of bereaved, 178, 185–86, 188, 190, 191
Transcendental meditation, 148
Treatment, 29–32, 102; continuous, 81
Treatment decisions, 5
Treatment terms (in General Systems Theory), 9–10, 11–12
Triazolam (Halcion), 193
Tricyclic antidepressants, 11, 21, 20, 42, 54, 55, 140, 195; in treatment of depression in conjugal bereavement, 200–9; in treatment of mourning, 192
Trimethobenzamide, 161
Trimethobenzamine, HCL, 133
Tryptophane, 25
Tupin, J. P., 55
Turnbull, F., 71
Twycross, R. G., 81, 111, 114, 118, 123, 125, 128, 129, 139
Tylenol, 160

Undermedication, 35, 79, 106
United Kingdom: treatment for bereaved in, 177–78
U.S. Department of Justice, 23
University of Rochester, 140, analgesic efficacy questionnaire, 130, 131T
Uremia, 161
Urine, 48, 49

Valentine, Amy, 129

Valium, 161
Value system(s), 3, 11–12, 13–14;
    internalized, 8; of treatment team, 10
Van Dyke, C., 137
Vasopressin, 170
Verebely, K., 121
Viola, A., 187
Violence, 4
Visitors, 20
Visual cortex, 170
Vitamin D metabolites, 114
Volkan, V., 187
Voluntary societies, 22
Von Bertalanffy, L., 5

Wahl, C. W., 189, 203
Wald, S. J., 111, 123
Walker, W. L., 185
Waltzmann, S., 203, 204

Wardlaw, S. L., 171
Warfarin, 44, 45
Warren, R. D., 55
Wayne County, Mich., 61
Weight loss, 20, 65, 200, 201, 205
Widows, 187, 188, 190, 192, 193, 201,
    206–8; grief stages in, 201–2
Wiener, A., 187, 189
Williams, B. A., 37
Withdrawal symptoms, 25, 99
Witkin, H. A., 69
Working through, 182

Yamamoto, T., 190
Young, M., 194

Zborowski, M., 67
Zilboorg, G., 4
Zung Depression Scale, 57

LIST OF CONTRIBUTORS

Editors

Ivan K. Goldberg, M.D., Associate in Clinical Psychiatry, Department of Psychiatry, College of Physicians and Surgeons, Columbia University
Sidney Malitz, M.D., Professor of Clinical Psychiatry, Department of Psychiatry, College of Physicians and Surgeons, Columbia University
Austin H. Kutscher, D.D.S., Professor of Dentistry (in Psychiatry), Department of Psychiatry, College of Physicians and Surgeons, Columbia University; Professor of Dentistry (in Psychiatry), Division of Oral and Maxillofacial Surgery, School of Dental and Oral Surgery, Columbia University; President, The Foundation of Thanatology

Contributors

David M. Benjamin, Ph.D., Department of Medical Research, Hoffmann-La Roche, Inc., Nutley, New Jersey
Richard S. Blacher, M.D., Clinical Professor of Psychiatry and Lecturer in Surgery, Tufts New England Medical Center, Boston, Massachusetts
Daniel Carr, M.D., Assistant Professor of Medicine (Endocrine Unit), Harvard Medical School and Massachusetts General Hospital, Boston, Massachusetts
Ching-Piau Chien, M.D., Department of Psychiatry, Albany Medical Center, Albany, New York
Bruce L. Danto, M.D., Fullerton, California; formerly, Director, Suicide Prevention Center, Detroit Psychiatric Institute, Detroit, Michigan
Wayne O. Evans, Ph.D., Massachusetts College of Pharmacy, Boston, Massachusetts
Irwin M. Greenberg, M.D., D.M. Sc., Medical Director, Jackson Brook Institute, South Portland, Maine
Balu Kalayam, M.D., Department of Psychiatry, Albany Medical Center, Albany, New York

M. Keeri-Szanto, M.D., Department of Anaesthesia, Victoria Hospital, London, Ontario, Canada

Robert Kellner, M.D., Ph.D., Professor, Department of Psychiatry, University of New Mexico School of Medicine; Chief, Psychiatry Service, Veterans Administration Hospital, Albuquerque, New Mexico

Samuel C. Klagsbrun, M.D., Associate Clinical Professor of Psychiatry, Department of Psychiatry, College of Physicians and Surgeons, Columbia University, New York, New York; Medical Director, Four Winds Hospital, Katonah, New York

Lillian G. Kutscher, Publications Editor, The Foundation of Thanatology, New York, New York

Patricia Murray, Ph.D., R.N., Counseling Associates, Staten Island, New York

Philip R. Muskin, M.D., Assistant Clinical Professor of Psychiatry, Department of Psychiatry, College of Physicians and Surgeons, Columbia University, New York, New York

Richard T. Rada, M.D., Department of Psychiatry, University of New Mexico School of Medicine, Albuquerque, New Mexico

William Regelson, M.D., Professor of Medicine, Medical College of Virginia, Virginia Commonwealth University, Richmond, Virginia

Arthur Rifkin, M.D., Department of Psychiatry, College of Physicians and Surgeons, Columbia University, New York, New York

Anthony F. Santore, A.C.S.W., Northwest Center for Community Mental Health/Mental Retardation Program, Philadelphia, Pennsylvania

Irene B. Seeland, M.D., Assistant Clinical Professor of Psychiatry, Department of Psychiatry, College of Physicians and Surgeons, Columbia University, New York, New York

Reuben J. Silver, M.D., Department of Psychiatry, Albany Medical Center, Albany, New York

Arleen I. Skversky, Northwest Center for Community Mental Health/Mental Retardation Programs, Philadelphia, Pennsylvania

Steven Steckel, Pharmacist, Strong Memorial Hospital, Rochester, New York

Richard F. Tislow, M.D., Department of Psychiatry, University of Pennsylvania; Northwestern Institute of Psychiatry; Northwest Center for Community Mental Health/Mental Retardation Programs, Philadelphia, Pennsylvania

Robert G. Twycross, M.A., D.M., F.R.C.P., Consultant Physician, Sir Michael Sobell House, The Churchill Hospital, Headington, Oxford, England

Amy Valentine, R.N., Strong Memorial Hospital, Rochester, New York

Michael Weintraub, M.D., Associate Professor in Preventive, Family, and Rehabilitation Medicine; Associate Professor of Pharmacology and Medicine, University of Rochester School of Medicine and Dentistry, Rochester, New York

Walter W. Winslow, M.D., Department of Psychiatry, University of New Mexico School of Medicine, Albuquerque, New Mexico

Stewart G. Wolf, M.D., Professor of Medicine, Temple University School of Medicine, Philadelphia, Pennsylvania; Director, Totts Gap Institute for Human Ecology, Bangor, Pennsylvania

Irving S. Wright, M.D., M.A.C.P., F.R.C.P., Emeritus Clinical Professor of Medicine, Cornell University Medical College, New York, New York; Past President, American College of Physicians; Past President, American Heart Association; Past President, American Geriatrics Society

COLUMBIA UNIVERSITY PRESS/ FOUNDATION OF THANATOLOGY SERIES

Teaching Psychosocial Aspects of Patient Care
Bernard Schoenberg, Helen F. Pettit, and Arthur C. Carr, editors

Loss and Grief: Psychological Management in Medical Practice
Bernard Schoenberg, Arthur C. Carr, David Peretz, and Austin H. Kutscher, editors

Psychosocial Aspects of Terminal Care
Bernard Schoenberg, Arthur C. Carr, David Peretz, and Austin H. Kutscher, editors

Psychosocial Aspects of Cystic Fibrosis: A Model for Chronic Lung Disease
Paul R. Patterson, Carolyn R. Denning, and Austin H. Kutscher, editors

The Terminal Patient: Oral Care
Austin H. Kutscher, Bernard Schoenberg, and Arthur C. Carr, editors

Psychopharmacologic Agents for the Terminally Ill and Bereaved
Ivan K. Goldberg, Sidney Malitz, and Austin H. Kutscher, editors

Anticipatory Grief
Bernard Schoenberg, Arthur C. Carr, Austin H. Kutscher, David Peretz, and Ivan K. Goldberg, editors

Bereavement: Its Psychosocial Aspects
Bernard Schoenberg, Irwin Gerber, Alfred Wiener, Austin H. Kutscher, David Peretz, and Arthur C. Carr, editors

The Nurse as Caregiver for the Terminal Patient and His Family
Ann M. Earle, Nina T. Argondizzo, and Austin H. Kutscher, editors

Social Work with the Dying Patient and the Family
Elizabeth R. Prichard, Jean Collard, Ben A. Orcutt, Austin H. Kutscher, Irene B. Seeland, and Nathan Lefkowitz, editors

Home Care: Living with Dying
Elizabeth R. Prichard, Jean Collard, Janet Starr, Josephine A. Lockwood, Austin H. Kutscher, and Irene B. Seeland, editors

Psychosocial Aspects of Cardiovascular Disease: The Life-Threatened Patient, the Family, and the Staff
James Reiffel, Robert DeBellis, Lester C. Mark, Austin H. Kutscher, Paul R. Patterson, and Bernard Schoenberg, editors

Acute Grief: Counseling the Bereaved
Otto S. Margolis, Howard C. Raether, Austin H. Kutscher, J. Bruce Povers,
Irene B. Seeland, Robert DeBellis, and Daniel J. Cherico, editors

The Human Side of Homicide
Bruce L. Danto, John Bruhns, and Austin H. Kutscher, editors

Hospice U.S.A.
Austin H. Kutscher, Samuel C. Klagsbrun, Richard J. Torpie, Robert DeBellis,
Mahlon S. Hale, and Margot Tallmer, editors

The Child and Death
John E. Schowalter, Paul R. Patterson, Margot Tallmer, Austin H. Kutscher,
Stephen V. Gullo, and David Peretz, editors

The Life-Threatened Elderly
Margot Tallmer, Elizabeth R. Prichard, Austin H. Kutscher, Robert DeBellis,
Mahlon S. Hale, and Ivan K. Goldberg, editors

Bei Fragen zur Produktsicherheit wenden Sie sich bitte an:
If you have any questions regarding product safety,
please contact:

Walter de Gruyter GmbH
Genthiner Straße 13
10785 Berlin
productsafety@degruyterbrill.com